Clinical Examination
of the Patient

Clinical Examination of the Patient

John S P Lumley,
MS, FRCS
Professor of Vascular Surgery
St Bartholomew's Hospital Medical School
London, UK

Pierre-Marc G Bouloux,
BSc, MD, FRCP
Senior Lecturer (Endocrinology)
Royal Free Hospital Medical School
London, UK

Photography by
Carole Reeves
MSc, FBIPP, FIMI

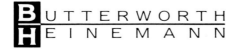

BUTTERWORTH
HEINEMANN

Butterworth-Heinemann Ltd
Linacre House, Jordan Hill, Oxford OX2 8DP

ℛ A member of the Reed Elsevier group

OXFORD   LONDON   BOSTON
MUNICH   NEW DELHI   SINGAPORE   SYDNEY
TOKYO   TORONTO   WELLINGTON

First published 1994

© Butterworth-Heinemann Ltd 1994

British Library Cataloguing in Publication Data
A catalogue record for this book is
available from the British Library

Library of Congress Cataloguing in Publication Data
A catalogue record for this book is
available from the Library of Congress

ISBN 0 7506 1671 7

Printed in Spain by Printeksa

Contents

Introduction

Clinical diagnosis and the assessment of the severity of disease are based on history, examination and investigation: the skillful acquisition of these three sources of information is thus essential to all clinicians. This atlas provides guidance on the three areas, with particular emphasis on the techniques of clinical examination.

The prime audience is the medical undergraduate starting clinical studies, but the student continually needs to perfect clinical skills and to prove competence in the final examination. In the latter, students can expect to be observed examining patients, and these conditions test the security of clinical examination to its full extent. It has been our experience that postgraduate students also need careful reappraisal of their techniques of clinical assessment before presenting themselves to higher examining authorities. It is our aim to provide a reliable yet flexible method of clinical assessment, appropriate to life-long professional application.

The component parts of a full history are outlined, together with the questions referrable to abnormalities of each system. The skilled clinician becomes an expert on the pattern recognition of diseases but the greatest skill is to listen to what the patient volunteers. This is the key to the diagnosis and the clinician must not shape, elaborate, flavour or direct a history into a particular category just so that it fits a classical package. Such prompting may result in mis-diagnosis.

Colour photographs are used to demonstrate clinical examination, with emphasis on the anatomy of the normal individual. The common variations of normality are highlighted, particularly in relation to differences of age, sex and race, increasing the awareness of the range of normality and facilitating its interpretation.

Disease represents loss or modification of function and a key feature of the examination is to ask the patient to demonstrate these abnormalities. Emphasis must be given to this factor in both history and examination. Be aware that the full house of classical physical signs of a specific disease are not present in every patient.

The purpose of an assessment is usually to identify abnormality and, although this text is concerned with examination techniques and the limits of normality, no excuse is made for introducing disease terminology. A glossary is included to define these terms, but the reader should use a companion volume, such as the author's edition of Hamilton Bailey's Physical Signs, for further study.

Pathological signs are only included when they provide the most satisfactory method of demonstrating specific examination techniques; no attempt has been made to produce a text of abnormal physical signs.

In a well perfected system of examination, the observer usually passes from the hands to the head and then down to the toes. However, the effect of disease is usually predominant in one body system and the initial sections are organized by system. Although the information presented provides a useful, logical way of diagnosis, there must be flexibility and adaptability to modify this approach to match a patient's presenting pathology. Every student is encouraged to develop his/her own method of assessment, based on the guidelines provided in this text.

The text is intended as a companion rather than a surrogate to bedside assessment. Most of the techniques described may be practised by students on themselves or colleagues, possibly under the supervision of a clinical teacher, before approaching a patient. Demonstration of the instruments of examination are limited to those which every clinician should carry or those routinely available on wards and in outpatient departments.

Investigations included are those commonly used to assess each system. These are, however, likely to become dated by technical and scientific advances, and should be taken only as a basic guide to this area of assessment.

The section on skills and attitudes in undergraduate medical education has been included to introduce the student to these topics early in his/her clinical training. The lists of competencies that should be acquired during the undergraduate course will serve as a checklist if no log book is provided.

Reference tables are included for comparing body segments, weights, heights and notes on neonatal screening and milestones. An additional section is included on patient note-keeping. Students should also consider how to file patient records, allowing subsequent retrieval by specific disease, symptom or sign. The chosen system must be compatible with life-long study of all aspects of patient management.

Skills and Attitudes in Undergraduate Medical Education

The principal function of undergraduate medical education is to prepare the student to assume the responsibility of a House Officer appointment. During the latter, supervision and training continue, until full registration brings the moral and legal obligations, and the responsibilities of independent patient management.

The development of professional attitudes appropriate to these responsibilities is a continuous process, during which every student must set personal standards of learning and other activities. External standards will be laid down, but these form only a basic core and should not limit one's horizons.

Personal standards and responsibilities to patients go far beyond a 9 to 5 business arrangement. Such committment requires the acquisition of appropriate knowledge and skills, and the setting of personal attitudes and ethical codes. Medical professionalism has to be based on a clear understanding of the process of patient management.

This chapter lists some of the skills that a patient could reasonably expect of a junior doctor. Young trainees would not necessarily be expected to undertake all the items in these lists unaided, but they should be confident that they understand what is involved.

Clinical Skills

Patient assessment by history, examination and appropriate investigations. Screening where necessary.

Interpretation of history, examination and investigations.

Problem solving.

Effective use of hospital and social services.

Knowledge of scientific, clinical and other resources.

Communication Skills

Discussing difficult problems with patients, particularly relating to serious illness, bad news and those of a sexual nature.

Discussion of management problems with a patient's relatives, bereavement counselling and organ donation.

Discussion of management problems with nurses, peers, seniors and other health care workers.

Organisational Skills

Patient management.

Links with hospital service departments: haematology, biochemistry, microbiology, histopathology, autopsy, radiology, pharmacy.

Support, development and other contributions to team activities and relationships.

Personal Development

Developing knowledge: through information gathering, library visits and preparation for undergraduate and postgraduate examinations.

Attending meetings: clinical, radiological, clinicopathological, death and complications, audit and journal clubs.

Presentations at clinical and other meetings.

Clerical Skills

Recording and updating patient records, filling out and following up investigation forms and their results.

Doctor's letters, discharge letters, summaries.

Issuing death certificates and reporting deaths to the coroner where appropriate.

Undertaking Audit

Structure, process and outcome measure of the clinical and managerial components of patient management.

Cost-effective management, cost-containment, the financial implications of various therapeutic procedures.

Preventive Medicine and Health Promotion

Advice on cigarettes, alcohol, recreational drugs, condoms, self-examination (breast and scrotum), diet and exercise.

Ethical and Legal Implications

Acquisition of appropriate knowledge to develop personal views and responsibility.

The following lists indicate the practical procedures and the management problems which will be encountered by the experienced medical student and junior doctor. They will not necessarily see or be involved in all of these activities as a junior, but every junior doctor must be aware of the management regime and be capable of undertaking these practical procedures in an emergency. In many cases it will be as a junior member of a resuscitation team.

Practical Procedures

Insertion of intravenous, central venous pressure and intra-arterial lines.

Taking venous and arterial blood for gas analysis.

Delivery of intravenous drugs, such as cytotoxics.

Recording and interpreting an electrocardiogram.

Pleural aspiration/biopsy; insertion of chest drain.

Passing nasogastric and orogastric tubes.

Stoma management; paracentesis; proctoscopy.

Male, female and suprapubic urinary catheterisation.

Unblocking urinary catheters, bladder irrigation and washouts.

Excision of skin lesions; wound suture and removal of sutures; management of drains.

Aspiration of cysts and abscesses.

Application and removal of plaster casts; skin traction; joint aspiration.

Management of Medical and Surgical Emergencies

Left ventricular failure, myocardial infarct, cardiac arrhythmias.

Cardiac arrest: DC shock, intracardiac puncture, external cardiac massage.

Cardio-pulmonary resuscitation.

Acute asthma/respiratory failure; mouth to mouth respiration and tracheal intubation.

Acute anaphylaxis.

Arterial embolism; ruptured abdominal aortic aneurysm.

Dysphagia, acute abdominal pain, intestinal obstruction, perforation of abdominal viscera, peritonitis, faecal impaction.

Strangulated inguinal hernia; appendicitis, diverticulitis, cholecystitis, salpingitis; ectopic pregnancy.

Acute/chronic urinary retention; haematuria, renal colic, urinary tract infection.

Testicular pain, torsion, epididymo-orchitis; priapism, phimosis, paraphimosis.

Injuries: acute haemorrhage, soft tissue, nerve, tendon; hand.
Fractures, dislocations.
Head, spinal, chest, abdomen.
Urinary tract, kidney, bladder, urethra.
Multiple injury.
Infection: hands, feet, abscesses, pyrexia, septicaemia.
Management of pain
Postoperative complications: wound, respiratory, airway, cardiorespiratory, deep vein thrombosis, pulmonary embolism, fluid balance.
Acute confusional/psychiatric states.
Subarachnoid haemorrhage, meningitis, status epilepticus.
Coma; overdoses, drug abuse.
Hypo/hyperkalaemia and calcaemia.
Diabetic ketosis, hypoglycaemia.
Acute renal failure.
Acute hepatic failure.
Terminal care.

Observe/Assisted/Undertaken

Biopsy: surgical/radiological of marrow, bone, liver, kidney.
Craniotomy; thoracotomy; laparotomy.
Scopes: bronchoscopy, mediastinoscopy, pleuroscopy, oesophagoscopy, gastro/duodenoscopy, retrograde hepatobiliary, sigmoidoscopy, colonoscopy, laparoscopy.
Arteriographic procedures: percutaneous transluminal angioplasty.
Barium studies; transhepatic biliary procedures.
A full range of surgical procedures.

Personal Development

The above lists of skills may seem rather daunting. However, when they are spread over a studentship and the first year pre-registration house appointments, all are achievable, and have already been achieved by the vast majority of one's predecessors.

Self-assessment is an important aspect of this development. As an individual knows more about him/herself and his/her limitations than anyone else, it is wise to document personal activities, experience and achievements, and to monitor progress. If the training scheme does not provide a log book, the above lists form an appropriate starting point to develop one's own.

Invite, and benefit from, peer review and discuss assessments with senior members of staff. They in turn will often be asked for reviews and references by the medical school or appointment committees.

When formulating such references, they will take into account:

A trainee's clinical judgment and skills; their concern for patients; responsibility, reliability and enthusiasm; health and punctuality; the ability to handle and withstand stress; their insight and acceptance of constructive criticism; keeping abreast of meetings and audit activities; their relation to patient's relatives, nurses, doctors and all members of staff; their contribution to team organisation, planning and functioning.

In conclusion, references will comment on a trainee's potential. In medicine, as in all branches of life, it is important that individuals match their aims and aspirations to their potential knowledge, skills and ability.

Postgraduate medical education merges into lifelong continuing medical education. This should not be looked on as a chore, but part of a desire to remain abreast of current practice. In this way, an individual can be assured, at least in their own mind, that they are providing optimal patient care, and having the satisfaction of achieving their maximum potential.

History Taking

A patient usually comes to a doctor with a specific problem (symptom) and the doctor's aim is to make the patient better. To do this he/she tries to work out what is causing the problem (diagnosis), determine its severity (assessment) and then institute appropriate treatment. The total process of assessment and treatment is termed management.

To diagnose and assess a patient's problems, the doctor can obtain information from three sources:
a) take a history
b) carry out a physical examination
c) request appropriate investigations

Although it is sometimes not possible to make a diagnosis, the process of assessment will often serve to exclude serious causes, allowing the doctor to reassure the patient and advise symptomatic treatment. It will also allow decisions to be made on follow-up and long term care. The following scheme for history taking is intended as an introduction to the subject, and outlines the prime headings that need to be considered when interviewing each patient.

Scheme for History Taking

First record the date of the examination. Note the patient's name, age, sex, occupation (past and present) and marital status (including any children).

The history emerges from the patient's description of the problem, directed by planned questioning. It is conveniently recorded under the following 6 sections.

SECTION 1: Present Illness

Presenting Complaint(s)

What brought the patient to hospital.

This must be put in a short statement, preferably in the patient's own words: for example, complaining of: 'abdominal pain and vomiting for the last 24 hours'; 'increasing breathlessness for 2 weeks'. If there is more than one complaint, these are listed and then they are taken in turn through the following.

History of Present Complaint(s)

This should record details of each problem, using mainly the patient's own words. Record as accurately as possible how long the complaint has been present and include the sequence of events in chronological order, with dates (e.g., one year ago, one month ago, yesterday). Let the patient begin by telling the story in their own words without interrupting. Afterwards, ask specific questions, using terms readily understood by the patient, either enlarging upon or clarifying their symptoms.

The presenting disorder is usually related to one system and questions referable to this, and any other system involved in the presenting complaint, are delivered at this stage (these questions are listed in Section 6). Pain is one of the most common symptoms and appropriate questions are given on page 18. Many of these questions can also be applied to other symptoms.

If the patient is a poor historian, unable to give a history, or one suspects is giving unreliable information, it may be helpful to talk to relatives or witnesses. Record the source of this and all aspects of the history which are not directly from the patient.

Previous History of Present Complaint(s)

If the patient has had similar symptoms in the past, give detailed information in chronological order, including any treatment received and the results of any investigations (if known). Report any past event with a clear bearing on the present condition, such as operations, trauma, weight loss, medication, contact with disease or recent travel abroad.

SECTION 2: Past Medical History

Note all other previous non-trivial illnesses, operations, accidents and periods of admission to hospital, not obviously related to the presenting condition, together with their dates.

Note illnesses, investigations, and immunizations in children. In adults, note relevant childhood problems, for example chronic respiratory disease, cardiac problems and rheumatic fever.

SECTION 3: Drugs and Allergies

Note all drugs being taken and their doses, and for how long they have been taken. What drugs have been taken in the past. Drug allergies: if allergic, what is meant by this term.

SECTION 4: Social and Personal History

Note current smoking habit, the number of years smoking and changes over this time. Note the usual alcohol consumption in units/day or week, and what is drunk: question whether the subject has ever been a heavy drinker. Ask whether any recreational drugs are used.

Record details of work and, where relevant, any difficulties with job, family or finances. Note any recent mental stress or problems with sleeping pattern. Does the patient live alone. On which floor. Are there lifts. Is the lavatory on a different floor. Are friends or relatives nearby. Do they receive or need home help or meals on wheels. Will the patient be able to return to previous residence and/or employment.

SECTION 5: Family History

Enquire of the state of health or cause of death of the patient's parents, siblings, other close relatives and spouse. Question whether any members of the family are suffering, or have suffered from the presenting condition(s). It often helps to draw a family tree.

SECTION 6: Systems Review

The history of the present complaint encompasses a detailed enquiry of at least one of the systems of the body: this part of the history reviews the remaining systems for unsuspected abnormalities. It is carried out using specific questions pertinent to each system. These are listed in note form in the following paragraphs and are further considered with the examination of each system. Non-specific symptoms may also be present, such as fever, lassitude, malaise and weight change.

Pain

Pain is frequently a presenting symptom in every system and the questions asked should include:
1. Where is the pain (site, focal, diffuse, radiation, referred).
2. When did the pain start—how often did it occur and how long did it last, was it sudden or gradual in onset or offset, and is it continuous, intermittent or fluctuating.
3. What is it like—in terms of severity, type (stabbing, aching, burning) and any systemic affects (nausea, vomiting, sweating, loss of sleep).
4. What makes the pain better (food, rest, posture, medication).
5. What makes the pain worse (food, coughing, posture).
6. What do you do during the attack.

It is worth studying these questions and reshuffling them into a form which one can easily remember, perhaps converting them into an acronym or an anagram.

Cardiovascular and Respiratory Systems

In the cardiovascular system consider the three areas of the body that are commonly affected: the heart, the brain (p 21) and the lower limbs, and the main risk factors: smoking, diabetes, hypertension, raised serum lipids and family history.

Pain

Cardiac pain: angina, on exercise or at rest, current or previous myocardial infarction. Site, radiation to neck or arm, accentuation by coughing.

Leg pain: intermittent claudication (pain on exercise), duration, distance, hills, number of stairs. Pain at rest, associated ulceration or gangrene

Palpitations (Awareness of Heart Beat)

At rest, how often, length and duration. Regular or irregular. Associated symptoms such as syncope (fainting).

Dyspnoea (Breathlessness)

At rest. When lying flat (orthopnoea), how many pillows used to sleep. Awaking breathless (paroxysmal nocturnal dyspnoea); on exercise (dressing, walking, climbing stairs, how far, how many). Wheezing, hayfever, bronchitis, pleurisy, tuberculosis. Date of last chest X-ray.

Cough

Dry or productive. If productive, appearance of the sputum: mucus, pus, haemoptysis (blood-stained, pure blood), and the amount.

Upper Respiratory Tract Infection

Nasal discharge, pain over sinuses, earache, sore throat. Cervical lymph node enlargement.

Peripheral Oedema (Fluid in Tissues)

Swelling of ankles, degree, constant or only in the evenings.
Varicose veins, venous thrombosis.

Alimentary System

Abdominal Pain (p 18)

Site, onset, colic, radiation to back, relation to food.

Weight Loss, Loss of Appetite

Heartburn, Indigestion, Flatulence

These are vague terms but are often used by the patient. If properly
analysed they may lead to some useful information.

Vomiting

With or without preceding nausea. Frequency. Time in relation to
meals. Appearance: clear, colour, undigested food, bile, blood.

Dysphagia (Difficulty in Swallowing)

Painful or painless. For solid food, fluids, or both. Where does the
food get stuck. Regurgitation (as opposed to vomiting).

Jaundice (Bile Colouring)

Degree (sclera, skin, dark urine, pale stool).

Distention or Localised Abdominal Swelling

Disturbances of Bowel Habit

The term constipation may be used to describe changes in bowel
habit, frequency of bowel action or hard stools—question all factors.
Number of evacuations per day. Diarrhoea. Features of stool (colour,
formed, loose, liquid, blood on it, blood mixed with it, mucus, pus).
Tenesmus (false desire to defecate). Pain on defecation. Discharge per rectum. Pruritus ani (itching). Perianal lumps—on straining, persistent,
painful.

Genitourinary System

Disturbances of Micturition

Urine: clear, discoloured, cloudy, blood stained. Polyuria. Frequency: day, night (nocturia). Dysuria (pain or burning on micturition). Difficulty in initiating stream. Poor stream. Post-micturition dribbling, urgency, tenesmus (false desire), incontinence. Urethral discharge (features).

Disturbances of the Female Genital System

Menstruation: frequency, duration, amount of blood lost, dysmenorrhea (pain). Age at menarche, pregnancies and complications, method of birth control, pill, menopause. Vaginal discharge (character). Dyspareunia (pain on intercourse), superficial or deep. Libido. Breasts: pain or lumps, nipple discharge (milk, blood, colour): self-examination.

Central Nervous System

Psychological, mental and personality changes. Disturbances of consciousness (how long, warning, what doing at the time, incontinence, associated injury, tongue biting). Associated features (such as chest pain, headache or palpitations). Disturbances of sleep. Disturbances of memory: recent events, past events. Headache. Motor disturbances—weakness, paralysis, abnormal movements, fits, faints, falls. Speech disturbances. Sensory deficits: paraesthesia (pins and needles), numbness, anaesthesia. Disturbances of the special senses: vision, hearing, smell, taste, balance.

Locomotor System and Joints

Trouble in limbs and spine: pain or limitation of movements of joints, stiffness, difficulty in use of joints. Swelling, wasting, contractures, deformity, limp.

Endocrine System
(See also Genitourinary System)

Weight loss or gain, heat/cold intolerance, diabetes, thirst, polyuria. Skin changes, pigmentation, hair loss. Voice changes, shaving, libido, potency, early morning erections. Are the subject's voice, facial and body hair, and breast size appropriate to their age and sex.

Dermatological System

Rashes or lumps: where. Onset: duration. Progress. Does it itch. Eczema, sensitivities. Changes in hair or nails.

Psychiatric Assessment

A psychiatric assessment follows a different format from that of the other systems. Emphasis is given to the mental state and the history predominates. However, a full systemic history and examination is still essential, and the following paragraphs indicate the *additional* information which is sought. Not all of this data is necessarily collected at the first or even subsequent interviews, but it serves as a guide to appropriate questioning.

The assessment starts with the *identification of the problem* and the *mode of referral*. This preliminary survey directs subsequent questioning. Next, define the *previous history*, establishing a basis on which to place the *present history*, and the *present mental and physical state*. The information may be obtained from a third party. The relationship of the informant must, however, be noted together with an impression of the reliability of the informant and of the information

Previous History

This includes questions on *family, personal, past medical and mental health*, and *previous personality*, providing an indication of how the patient was before the onset of the current illness.

Family History (Where Known)

Age, health, cause of death, personality and occupation of parents and siblings. History of mental illness, neuroses, epilepsy, suicides, alcoholism.

Quality of home atmosphere; influence of parents, parental and sibling relationships, and any continuing problems; material and environmental support.

Relation of family, genetic factors, environment or other problems, to the patient's illness.

Personal History

Date and place of birth.

Birth and early development: pregnancy, type of delivery, feeding; milestones for walking, talking, and bladder and bowel control.

Childhood behaviour, emotional maladjustment, tantrums, sleep walking, bedwetting, thumb sucking, nail biting, stammers, food fads.

Education

Age for reading, and starting and stopping school; relation to teachers and peers, nicknames, body build, ability at work and games, hobbies and interests, higher education, qualifications.

Occupation

List work chronologically: explain any interruptions. Job satisfaction, ambitions, wages. Military service: if so, where.

Social

Finances, housing, social group.

Sexual and Marital Adjustment (Education, Activities and Abuse)

Onset of puberty, menstrual history, commencement of sexual relationships, mode and frequency of sexual encounters, hetero/homosexual, masturbation, fetishes, premarital and extramarital relationships, contraception. Engagement length, marriage, marital relationships, attitude to pregnancy, abortions, stillbirths. Parenthood, children: age, development and relationships.

Previous Health

Physical Illnesses

Operations, accidents, other treatments and their influence on present complaint (list chronologically with dates and recovery time).

Psychiatric Disorders

Hysterical, preoccupations of body, insomnia, mood, obsessions, anxiety, tensions, psychosomatic (list chronologically with treatment and precipitating factors).

Previous Personality

(As described by the patient or, in cases of communication difficulties, from a named close associate)

Cognition: Intellect, achievement (do these equate to education—what does the patient think.)

Motivation: Energy, falling asleep.

Character: Impulsive, reserved.

Emotional state (affect): Changeable (rapid, slow), agressive, optimistic, anxious, self-concerned, depressed, suicidal.

Fantasy life: Daydreams and their content.

Habits: Food fads, sleeping habits, alcohol, smoking, over or under-weight.

Standards: Oral, social, religious; encounters with the law.

Social life and leisure activities : Choice of reading, TV, hobbies, interests.

Relationships: With family, friends and workmates.

Living arrangements: Who with.

History of Present Illness or Problems

Onset, development, frequency and duration of each psychological symptom or change in behaviour: description of severity, precipitating factors and treatment. Associated bodily symptoms (with location).

What events preceded or may have led to the current problems. Emotional upsets, social problems, changes, encounters, separation, conflict, change in lifestyle, physical change.

What are the consequences in personal relationships, marriage and family life, work, leisure interest, accommodation and finances.

Present State

Current Mental State

This assessment is based on observations made during history taking. Questions are introduced into natural conversation with minimal direct questioning. However, the record is written up in a structured format, avoiding vague, poorly defined terms. The information partly overlaps the history of the previous personality but this section represents the *interpretation by the examiner*, whereas the previous personality is based on the *opinion of the patient* or close associate. In particular, note recent changes related to the current illness. The list is not exhaustive; add further questions and reshuffle the order to make it easier to remember.

General Behaviour

Appearance (personal hygiene, grooming): relate to age, education and socioeconomic status.

Activity: abnormal movements.

Disturbances of Consciousness

Alert, confused, drowsy (can be fully aroused), stupor (cannot be fully aroused), light coma (cannot be aroused), deep coma (loss of reflexes).

Orientation

Knows date, time, place, and identity of self and examiner.

Emotional State (Mood)

How do you feel? Judged by expression and inflection of voice, gesture and habitus: labile, elated, flat, angry, agitated, anxious, afraid, depressed, suicidal.

Insight, Judgment

Understands nature of current problem, its origin and the need for treatment.

Thought (Spoken, Written) Process and Content

Amount (spontaneous, silent), rate, fluency.

Inappropriate content, repeating questions, perseveration (reworded response), neologism (making up words), and syntactical or semantic errors.

Organic disease may compromise the organization of language, and interpretation is made more difficult by disturbances of speech, writing, hearing, and disturbances of consciousness and memory.

Hallucinations

False impressions of special and somatic sensation.

Delusions and Misinterpretations

False beliefs.

Compulsive Phenomena and Obsessions

Cognitive and Intellectual Function

(i) *Attention and concentration*: interest in surroundings.

(ii) *Memory loss (amnesia)*: immediate recall, recent (within one hour), long term. Name of relatives, date of birth and address.

(iii) *Learning*: repeat immediately and after a short interval, 3 or 4 unrelated words, and 4 to 6 digits forwards and backwards.

(iv) *Calculation* (acalcuria): counting backwards from 100 by 3 or 7, simple addition and multiplication.

(v) *Apraxia* (cannot use objects), *Agnosia* (cannot recognise objects), recognision of sensations (e.g. objects seen, or felt), *Agraphia* (cannot write), *Alexia* (cannot read)

(vi) *General knowledge*: current events, sports, hobbies.

(vii) *Vocabulary*: relate to education.

(viii) *Reasoning*: interpretation of proverbs and similarities.

(ix) Intelligence testing.

Current Physical State

Physical disease causing mental impairment or interfering with the patient's way of life.

Unrelated current problems.

Physical Examination

When undertaking a physical examination, aim to keep the patient comfortable, relaxed and reassured. Talk through what is going to happen, if this is not obvious, and ensure minimal discomfort and inconvenience. A warm environment is essential and, similarly, the examiner's hands must be warm. The privacy of a small room or a curtained area is desirable, with optimal, preferably natural, lighting.

The patient undresses down to underclothes and puts on a dressing gown. He or she then lies supine on a couch, with an adjustable back to provide head support, covered with a sheet or blanket. Each area must be adequately exposed as required, without embarrassment to the patient. A chaperon may be appropriate when examining members of the opposite sex. Relatives are usually best excluded except when examining children.

The examiner stands on the right side of the patient. The order of examination is regional rather than by system, although the central nervous system is often examined as an entity, together with various parts of the locomotor system, at the end of the procedure.

It is usual to commence the examination with the hands and then to proceed methodically from head to toe, surveying all systems and later integrating these findings, as subsequent verbal presentations and recording in the notes are usually by system. Thoroughness is important: efficiency and speed develop with practice. The examination time should not be prolonged in ill or frail patients and in emergencies it may be appropriate to concentrate on diseased areas, completing a routine examination at a later time.

The text takes a regional approach in examination of the head and neck, chest and abdomen but links the chest to the cardiovascular and respiratory systems and the abdomen to the alimentary system. Notes on further areas of interest are added in each case. The neurological and locomotor systems are considered separately. Cross references are given where applicable to avoid repetition.

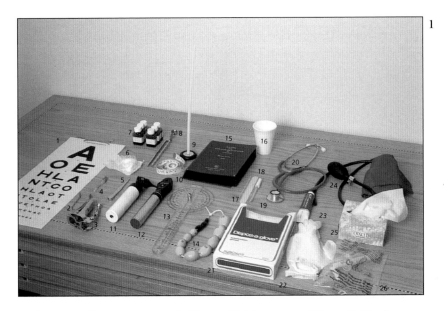

1 Common instruments carried by a clinician or readily available for out-patient or in-patient examination are demonstrated and listed.

1	Snellen chart	14	Beads for testicular sizing
2	Nasal speculum	15	Test charts for colour vision
3	Vaginal speculum	16	Cup
4	Sterile pin	17	Wooden stick
5	Two point retractor	18	Wooden spatula
6	Cotton wool	19	Thermometer
7	Bottles of odorants	20	Stethoscope
8	Tuning fork	21/	Disposable gloves
9	Patellar hammer	22	
10	Tape measure	23	Lubricant
11	Auroscope	24	Cuff of sphygmomanometer
12	Ophthalmoscope	25	Tissues
13	Goniometer	26	Disposable proctoscope

General Impression

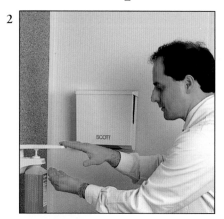

2 Washing hands—the examiner should wash hands before and after each patient examination and don gloves whenever mucous membranes are manually examined. Hand washing also allows the examiner to ensure he or she has warm hands at the beginning of each examination.

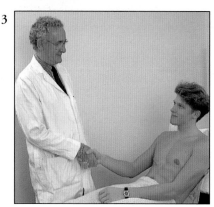

3 At the commencement of each history and examination the clinician introduces him- or herself to the subject, extending the appropriate national courtesies. The handshake demonstrated would usually be at the commencement of the history. The subject is in a closed, warm environment, stripped to the waist but covered with a blanket.

Throughout history taking the clinician is gaining an impression of the physical and mental status of the patient and the severity of his disability as well as attempting to make a diagnosis. Physical examination continues these observations, giving information on the patient's general state of health, his shape, posture, state of hygiene and mental and physical activity. Observe the exposed parts, particularly the hands, skin, head and neck.

The patient may be fit and well, but problems with diet or disease can lead to alteration of nutrition and hydration, such as obesity, weight loss, cachexia, loss of skin turgor and skin laxity.

Mental Status

A patient's behaviour may be influenced by the unaccustomed situation of being a patient, or by the effect of his disease, particularly if there is pain. This may be manifest by his facial expression, the degree of eye contact, restlessness, sweating, anxiety, apathy, depression, lack of cooperation or aggression. Note whether the patient's intelligence and personality equate to what one would expect from the history, or whether this could have changed in relation to the disease.

Drugs, head injuries and other diseases of the central nervous system can affect the level of consciousness, varying through alert, slow, confused, lacking concentration, and reduced level of response to spoken and physical stimuli. Impairment of motor function can produce weakness or spasticity. These may affect speech, posture, gait, and other movements, such as undressing. There may be added movements, such as tremor, or lack of coordination.

Abnormal Facies and Body Configuration

A number of congenital and endocrine diseases have characteristic general features amenable to spot diagnosis. However, one needs experience to differentiate between minor changes and the extremes of normality. Thus, be aware of the danger of jumping to false conclusions. Congenital examples are Down's, Turner's and Marfan's syndromes, achondroplasia and hereditary telangiectasia. Endocrine abnormalities include acromegaly, Cushing's disease, myxoedema and thyrotoxicosis. Other 'spot diagnoses' include Paget's disease and Parkinsonism.

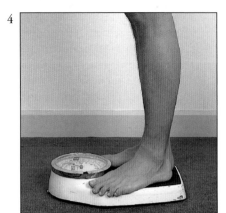

4 Weight—should be a routine assessment on the first out-patient visit and on admission to a ward; this serves as a baseline for subsequent progress of a disease or therapy.

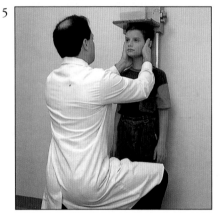

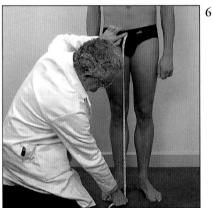

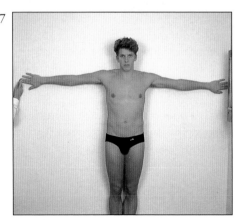

5 to 7 A subject can usually state his or her height but accurate assessment may be important when considering endocrine abnormalities, together with measurement of segments and span.

Charts

The charts at a patient's bed contain details of identification, such as name, date of birth, hospital number, ward and date, and commonly record temperature, pulse, respiratory rate, blood pressure, weight, bowel habit and the results of urine testing.

Urine testing and examination of any sputum or abnormal faeces are part of a routine patient examination.

The Hands

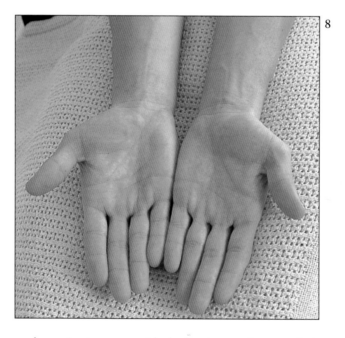
8

8 The general examination starts with the hands: sweating or soft tissue overgrowth may have been noted during the introductory handshake. Skin abnormalities of the palm and dorsum of the hands are usually easier to see in a white skinned individual. They include pallor, cyanosis, polycythemia, pigmentation, bruises, rashes and nicotine stains. The state of nutrition can be influenced by vascular insufficiency, and also by the patient's occupation. Liver disease can give rise to spider naevi and a characteristic palmar flushing. Dupuytren's contracture, nodules and moles are common findings.

Muscle wasting can be seen at an early stage in the small muscles of the hand, indicating a peripheral nerve injury or systemic disease. Muscle fasciculation or tremors may be present together with joint abnormalities, such as those of rheumatoid or osteoarthritis and acromegaly.

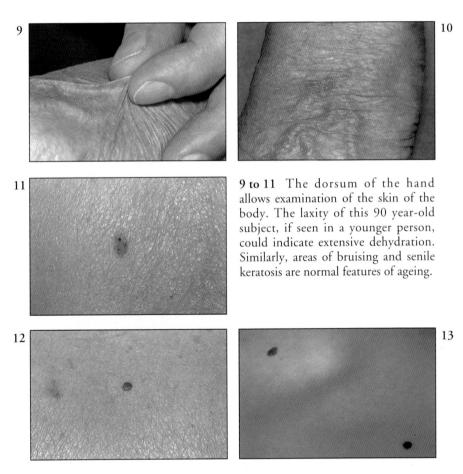

9 to 11 The dorsum of the hand allows examination of the skin of the body. The laxity of this 90 year-old subject, if seen in a younger person, could indicate extensive dehydration. Similarly, areas of bruising and senile keratosis are normal features of ageing.

12 and 13 Campbell de Morgan spots and moles are common normal findings.

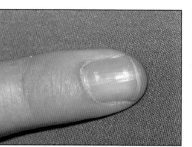

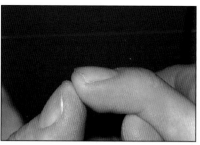

14 Nails may be brittle and deformed. White marks and ridges are common features associated with minor trauma, but may also indicate malnutrition. Pallor and cyanosis may be obvious. Note any spooning or splinter haemorrhages, indicative of systemic disease.

15 Look for the normal angle of the nail fold. Subungual swelling, arching of the nail and splaying of the distal phalanx indicate clubbing: compress the base of the nail to show the abnormal movement of the nail bed commonly present in this condition.

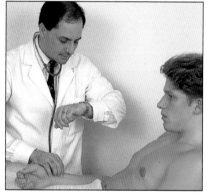

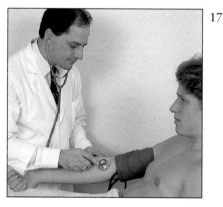

16 Examination of the pulse is considered in more detail under the Vascular System (p 68) but at this stage in the general examination it is counted for at least half a minute, and abnormalities of volume, character and rhythm noted.

17 This is a useful point to measure blood pressure, as it may be inadvertently omitted if not routinely positioned in the examination.

Blood Pressure

The upper limb is fully exposed, and the patient sits or lies on a couch. An appropriately sized blood pressure cuff must be used: in adults this is 12.5cm. It should not impinge on the axilla or the cubital fossa, and should be wrapped closely and evenly around the upper arm. Smaller cuffs are available for children. Too small a cuff can give a falsely high reading, while too large a cuff prevents access to the brachial artery. The manometer should be at the eye level of the observer.

The radial pulse is palpated as the cuff is inflated. The pressure is raised to approximately 30mmHg above the level at which the pulse disappears. A stethoscope is lightly applied over the brachial artery on the medial aspect of the cubital fossa and the cuff pressure lowered 5mmHg at a time. The systolic blood pressure is the level at which the sound is first heard. The diastolic is the point at which the sound becomes suddenly faint or inaudible (Korotkoff sounds I, IV, V—appearance, muffling, disappearance).

In cardiovascular disease, the blood pressure is taken in both arms and, in patients with treated or untreated hypertension, in lying and standing positions. If a patient is anxious, a falsely high reading may be obtained, together with an increased pulse rate. When abnormal readings are obtained, the recording should be repeated: the pressure in the cuff being allowed to drop to zero between measurements.

In peripheral vascular disease the blood pressure may also be measured in the lower limbs. A wider cuff is required for thigh compression, and a Doppler probe is used to detect the presence or absence of a distal pulse. The systolic blood pressure is the point of reappearance of audible pulsation when letting down the cuff.

The Head and Neck

Examination of the head and neck incorporates many overlapping systems. These include examination of the Cranial Nerves (p 143), the Ear, Nose and Throat (p 40), the Alimentary (p 108), Cardiovascular (p 66), Respiratory (p 92) and Musculo-skeletal (p 83) Systems. The Cervical Nodes are considered on p 48. There may also be enlargement of the Salivary (p 42) and Thyroid Glands (p 44).

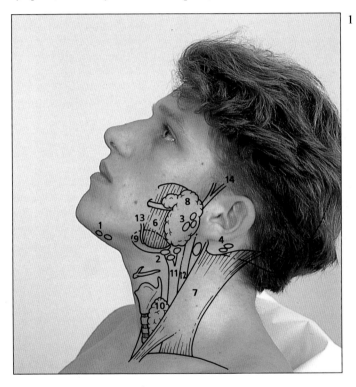

1

1 Lateral view of the head and neck, demonstrating lymph nodes, salivary and thyroid glands, the common carotid artery bifurcation and the internal jugular vein.

1	Submental lymph nodes	6	Masseter muscle
2	Submandibular lymph nodes	7	Sternomastoid muscle
3	Parotid lymph nodes	8	Parotid gland
4	Postauricular lymph nodes	9	Submandibular gland
5	Occipital lymph nodes	10	Thyroid gland

11	Common carotid artery
12	Internal jugular vein
13	Facial artery
14	Superficial temporal artery

Generalised weight loss may be apparent in changing facial and cervical contour. Excess tissue fluid (oedema) is subject to the effect of gravity and although mostly observed in the lower limbs towards the end of the day, it may also be obvious within the face, particularly the eyelids, after a night's sleep.

Whereas pallor and cyanosis of the hands may be due to the cold, these signs in the warm central areas of the lips and tongue may have more generalised significance, as does pallor.

2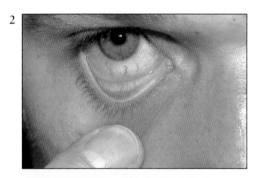

2 The pallor of anaemia is most noticeable on mucous membranes, although the sign lacks specificity. The inner surface of the lower lid is an important area for demonstration.

3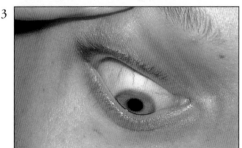

3 Mild degrees of jaundice are most easily picked up by staining of the sclera, producing a uniform colour change. Slight peripheral yellow discolouration is commonly seen in normal subjects.

4 Examine for evidence of pallor of mucous membranes, central cyanosis (particularly the tongue) abnormal pigmentation and dental hygiene. More details of examination of the , parotid and submandibular glands, and the teeth are considered on pages 42 and 109.

4

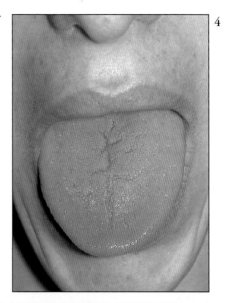

5

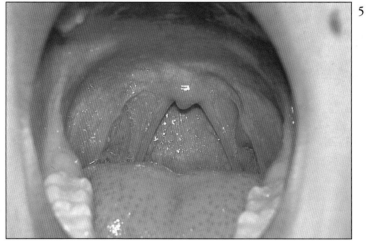

5 Note any furring of the tongue and inspect the tonsillar bed and the oropharynx for erythema. The tonsils and the lymphoid follicles on the back of the oropharynx are often prominent in young subjects.

The Ear, Nose and Throat

The tongue, floor of mouth and the oropharynx are considered in the General (p 39) and the Alimentary (p 108) Examinations. Abnormalities of the larynx, such as inflammation and neoplasia, may interfere with the airway and/or produce voice changes. Damage to the recurrent laryngeal nerve (p 44) may be produced by cancer of the thyroid, cervical oesophagus or the apex of the lung. The larynx may be observed by indirect laryngoscopy using a circular mirror, mounted on a long handle, rested on the soft palate. A head mirror is used to direct light through this mirror into the larygopharynx, in order to observe the entrance of the larynx and the vocal cords. A smaller mirror may be placed behind the palate to observe the posterior nares and the adenoids.

The nose is commonly damaged by direct trauma, and may be enlarged in acromegaly and myxoedema, or become reddened or enlarged in alcoholism. The commonest cause of nasal obstruction and discharge is infection, such as a cold, but foreign bodies, polyps and septal deviation are frequently encountered. Epistaxis (bleeding nose) may follow minor trauma; the bleeding point is usually anterior. The anterior part of the nose can be examined directly and this is facilitated by using a nasal speculum

1

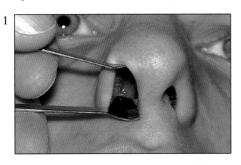

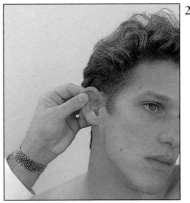

1 A nasal speculum is introduced antero-posteriorly to avoid stimulating the sensitive nasal septum. With the use of a head mirror, light may be directed into the anterior nares to observe the inferior concha, the anterior nasal cavity and the nasal septum.

2 Gentle pulling upwards and backwards of the auricle allows straightening of the external auditory meatus and the detection of abnormalities within the canal.

Deformities of the auricle, such as bat ears, are common and anomalies may be associated with syndromes such as Down's. Infection of the external auditory meatus (otitis externa) may produce pain and discharge; earache may also be referred from the teeth, temporomandibular joint, larygopharynx and cervical spine. Other symptoms of middle ear disease are deafness (see also p 151), tinnitus and vertigo, although these may occur in diseases of the central nervous, skeletal and cardiovascular systems, or with some drugs. Infection of the middle ear (otitis media) may produce redness and bulging of the eardrum. Extension of the infection into the mastoid air cells or the paranasal air sinuses may produce tenderness within the ear or over the cheeks and frontal region. Otitis media may be complicated by perforation of the tympanic membrane and damage to the ossicles.

3 A detailed view of the drum is provided with an auroscope, care being taken that the hand holding the instrument is also resting on the head so that any head movement by the subject carries no risk of the instrument being forced further into the canal.

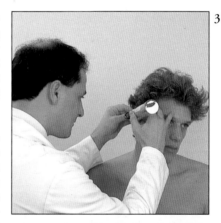

3

4 The tympanic membrane is translucent grey in the normal subject. It is oval in shape and lies obliquely, with its lateral surface facing downwards and forwards. The handle of the malleus is attached to the medial surface and can be seen through the drum, extending from the centre to the antero-superior flaccid part of the membrane. This part is limited by anterior and posterior folds radiating from the lateral process of the malleus.

The lower end of the handle of the malleus is firmly attached to the centre of the drum and at this point it produces a small elevation. On auroscopy a cone of light passes antero-inferiorly from the elevation. However, in this illustration, the right tympanic membrane has been photographed through an operating microscope and the cone is sited posteriorly.

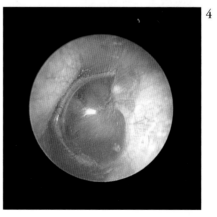

4

Salivary Glands

The large paired salivary glands (parotid, submandibular, submaxillary) are subject to generalised enlargement: this may be symmetrical, as in mumps, or variable as in sarcoid, and Sjörgen's and Mikulicz's syndromes. Like all glands, they are subject to inflammation and neoplasia, while blocking of a duct, by a stone or inspissated debris, may produce intermittent swelling on eating, and progress to retrograde infection and abscess formation. Swellings of the submandibular and parotid glands are easily mistaken for enlargement of the overlying lymph nodes.

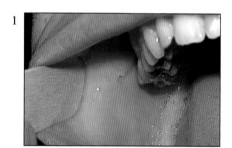

1 The parotid duct opens opposite the crown of the second upper molar tooth.

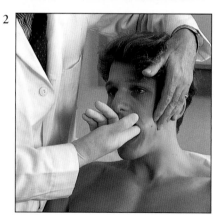

2 The parotid gland is palpated mainly externally but also bimanually around the anterior border of the ramus of the mandible. The gland extends below and behind the angle of the jaw and parotid lumps in this region may be difficult to differentiate from lymph nodes or submandibular enlargement.

3 The submandibular ducts open on the sublingual papillae on either side of the midline, adjacent to the frenulum of the tongue. Saliva can be seen to exude from the papillae and occasionally a submandibular calculus becomes lodged at this site.

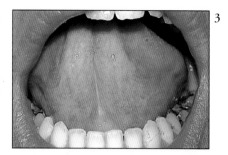

4 The sublingual and submandibular glands can be palpated bimanually throughout their lengths in the floor of the mouth.

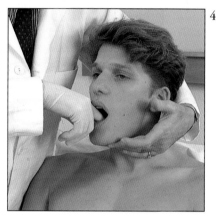

The Thyroid

Enlargement of the thyroid gland (goitre) is in the lower anterior part of the neck, partly covered by the sternomastoid muscles. The gland is attached to the larynx by fascial layers and therefore moves on swallowing. A goitre may involve the whole or only part of the gland and be of varying consistency. Diffuse enlargement may be physiological, due to deficiency problems or associated with thyrotoxicosis: a firm enlargement of the gland is seen in Hashimoto's disease. Nodules may be single or multiple: most are cysts, but more than 1 in 10 solitary nodules are malignant.

A goitre can compress the trachea causing airway obstruction. Damage to the recurrent laryngeal nerve (usually a sign of malignancy) will produce voice changes; vocal cord paralysis can be observed by indirect laryngoscopy (p 40). The increased metabolism of thyrotoxicosis is associated with many systemic symptoms and on examination there may be weight loss and a hyperactive state. Additional signs can be found in the eyes and hands (see below). Other thyroid related signs are the slow relaxation of tendon jerks and galactorrhoea found in myxoedema.

1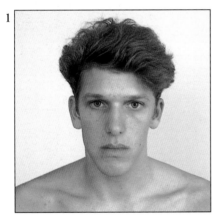

1 The subject is first observed from the front to define any obvious thyroid swelling (goitre) and note any asymmetry of the neck.

2 The thyroid is next observed during swallowing. The subject takes a mouthful of water, holds it, extends the neck and swallows when directed to by the examiner. The thyroid ascends with the larynx on swallowing and any enlargement is then more obvious.

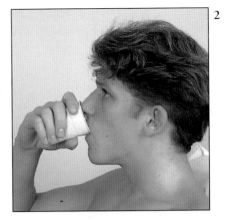

3 The lobes are more easily felt and compared with the examiner standing behind the subject. The isthmus is first palpated in the midline over the upper tracheal rings.

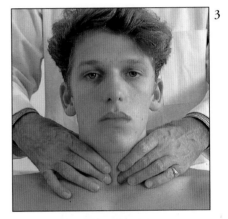

4 Each lobe is individually palpated. The subject flexes and rotates the neck towards the side of palpation, to relax the sternomastoid muscle. The non-palpating hand can be used to push the larynx to the opposite side and facilitate palpation, as seen in the next figure.

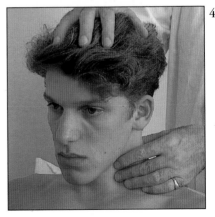

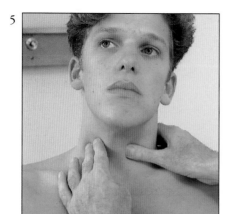

5 The lobes may also be palpated from in front. The larynx is again deviated from the opposite side, to push the lobe laterally against the examiner's fingers.

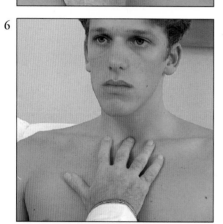

6 The position of the trachea is noted to define any deviation produced by asymmetrical thyroid enlargement.

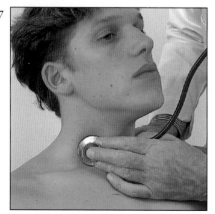

7 The lobes and isthmus are auscultated to pick up systolic and diastolic murmurs over a hyperaemic gland. The diaphragm of the stethoscope is lightly applied to avoid compression and artifactual production of murmurs from a carotid artery.

8 A large retrosternal goitre may have been detected rising out of the superior mediastinum on swallowing. It may also be detected by percussion over the manubrium.

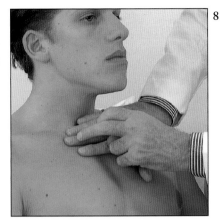

9 In thyrotoxicosis there may be lid retraction, lid lag and exophthalmos affecting eye movements. Lid lag is elicited by requesting the subject to follow a descending target, noting the delayed dropping of the upper lid. The imbalance produced by infiltration and fibrosis of the extraocular muscles may also give rise to abnormalities of gaze (p 146). Exophthalmos (protrusion of the eyeball) is most obvious when standing behind a sitting subject and looking downwards.

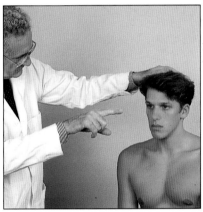

10 When examining the hands of a thyrotoxic subject there may be excess sweating, increased pulse rate and also a fine tremor, the latter can be highlighted by resting a sheet of paper on the dorsum of the outstretched hands.

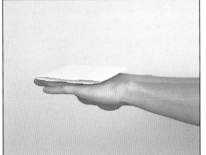

Cervical and Other Lymph Nodes

Cervical Nodes

The cervical lymph nodes are commonly enlarged, secondary to infective conditions of the tonsil, throat, ear and nose, and are the commonest lumps in the neck. They may occasionally undergo suppuration with abscess formation, this being more common with tuberculous lymphadenitis. Cervical node enlargement may also be the first sign of generalised lymphatic disease or of metastases.

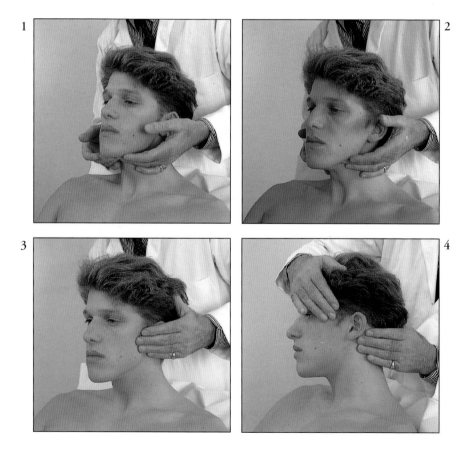

1 to 5 The submental, submandibular, parotid, postauricular and occipital nodes are examined in their circle around the base of the skull.

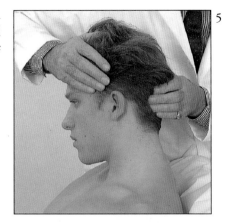

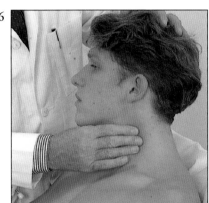

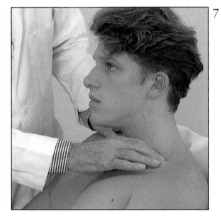

6 and 7 The deep cervical lymph chain, lying around the internal jugular vein commences in the submandibular triangle, passes deep to the sternomastoid muscle and extends laterally into the supraclavicular region.

8

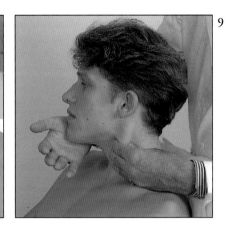

9

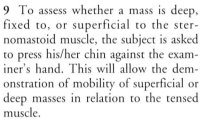

8 The scalene node can easily be missed if the examiner does not palpate deeply behind the lower end of the relaxed sternomastoid muscle.

9 To assess whether a mass is deep, fixed to, or superficial to the sternomastoid muscle, the subject is asked to press his/her chin against the examiner's hand. This will allow the demonstration of mobility of superficial or deep masses in relation to the tensed muscle.

10

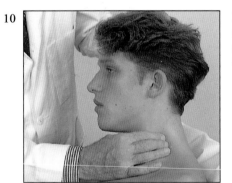

10 Smaller superficial nodes are frequently palpable along the line of the external, and to a lesser extent the anterior, jugular veins.

Having completed the examination of head and neck this is an opportune time to proceed to examination of the axillae and if enlarged nodes are located, also to examine for inguinal, epitrochlear and popliteal node enlargement and for hepatosplenomegaly (p 122/124). In practice, in the absence of suspected lymphadenopathy the axillary nodes in the female are examined with the breast and the thorax in the male. The inguinal nodes are palpated at the time of examination of the inguinal and scrotal regions.

Axillary Nodes (see also p 62)

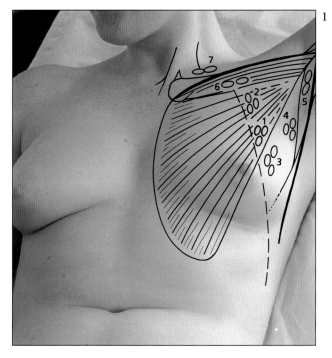

1   Lateral view of Axilla, demonstrating lymph node groups

1	Anterior	4	Posterior
2	Apical	5	Lateral
3	Medial	6	Infraclavicular
	7 Supraclavicular		

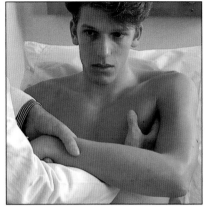

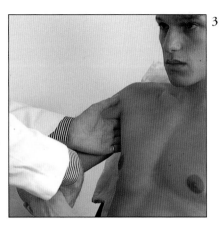

2 and 3 The examiner takes the weight of the arm when examining for axillary nodes. Anterior nodes are compressed against the anterior wall of the axilla.

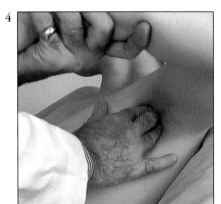

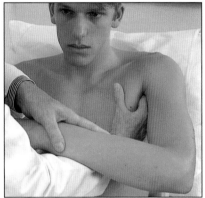

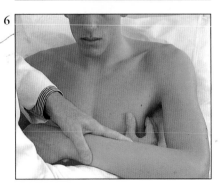

4 to 6 In the illustrations, the arm is raised to demonstrate the position of the cupped hand palpating the apical nodes. In practice, the arm is by the subject's side as the examining hand is drawn down over the medial axillary wall.

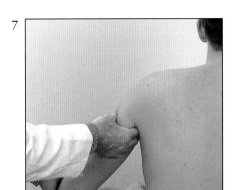 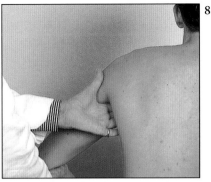

7 and 8 The lateral and posterior nodes are examined from behind.

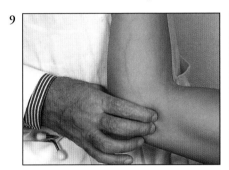 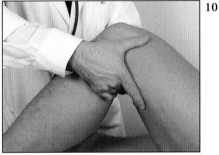

9 Epitrochlear nodes are palpated just above the medial epicondyle of the humerus.

10 Popliteal nodes may be palpable deeply placed over the popliteal vein in the lower aspect of the popliteal fossa.

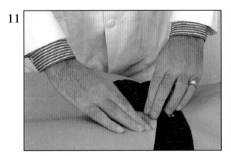 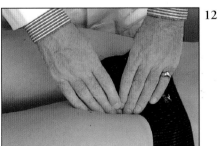

11 and 12 The horizontal group of inguinal nodes lie below and parallel to the inguinal ligament and the vertical group along the femoral vessels, in the centre of the femoral triangle. Inguinal nodes are commonly palpable in the normal subject.

Checklist for the Examination of the Head and Neck

Eye

Exophthalmos, enophthalmos, glaucoma

Conjunctiva: inflammation, chemosis, pallor, subconjunctival haemorrhage

Sclera: red, yellow, blue, brown

Cornea/lens: scars, abrasions, ulcer, cataract, arcus senilis, sclerolimbic calcification.

Movements: lid lag, ptosis, extraocular movements, nystagmus, fatiguability of pursuit movements

Facial palsy: upper/lower motor neurone

Visual fields: to confrontation with finger and white pin head

Visual acuity: Snellen's chart; reading chart

Fundi: optic disc, vessels, macula

Ear

Pinna: malformation; gouty tophi

External auditory meatus: wax; infection

Tympanic membrane; scarring, redness, perforation, bulging (and Valsalva)

Hearing: whisper; Rinne's and Weber's tests

Mouth

Lips: telangiectasia, swelling, ulceration, pigmentation, Koplik's spots

Gums: gingivitis, hypertrophy, retraction

Teeth: discoloration, caries, periodontal abscess

Tongue: glossitis, atrophy, macroglossia, geographic tongue, ulceration, leukoplakia, fetor

Tonsil: redness, purulent discharge

Oropharynx: redness, purulent discharge

Salivary glands: tenderness, swelling (abscess, cysts, tumours), duct calculi

Neck

Lymph nodes: submental, submandibular, preauricular, postauricular, occipital; deep and superficial cervical lymph chains

Trachea: midline, deviated

Thyroid: palpable, enlarged, symmetrical, focal lump (cyst, benign, malignant tumours), tracheal deviation, retrosternal extension, bruit

Carotid arteries: enlargement, bruits

The Female Breast and Axilla

A rise in public awareness of the need to treat early breast malignancy has prompted self-examination and attendance at screening programmes. Patients usually present with a lump, but pain and nipple discharge are important symptoms and may indicate underlying pathological changes.

Most lumps are benign and nodularity, discomfort and tenderness are common symptoms, often bilateral, and undergoing cyclical variation with menstruation. Take a full menstrual history, noting pregnancies, breast feeding, use of the pill and hormone replacement.

The patient should be asked about previous lumps, their management and any family history of breast malignancy. The most important genetic link is premenstrual malignancy in a first degree relative. A persistent or progressive lump requires further investigation, possibly with mammography or needle aspiration. Mammography can be diagnostic of benign or malignant disease while aspiration may eradicate a cyst and remove anxiety. Aspirate from solid lesions is examined histologically. A subsequent diagnosis of malignancy allows planned intervention, with patient involvement.

Progression of local malignancy will give rise to skin and deep tethering, nipple inversion and, when more extensive, skin ulceration. There may also be spread to local lymph nodes and metastases, particularly to bone, liver and lungs, these areas being a routine part of the physical examination of breast disease.

The commonest nipple discharge is milk and this may persist after pregnancy or present at other times (galactorrhoea), such as in endocrine abnormalities. Green or yellow discharge are often associated with cystic disease of the breast, blood staining may accompany benign or malignant lesions and the cause must always be identified.

Seclusion and warmth are particularly important in examination of the breast, to avoid discomfort and embarrassment to a patient. A good light is essential, to detect minor abnormalities.

There is wide variation in size, shape and consistency of the female breast, not only between individuals, but also within each subject during development, the menstrual cycle, pregnancy and in later life. If the breasts are asymmetrical establish if this is recent or longstanding.

The nipple usually points forward; unilateral or bilateral nipple retraction may be congenital, but recent changes and nipple deviation suggest underlying disease, as do a discharge or surrounding eczema. The initial pink coloured areolar becomes darker with age and brownish after pregnancy. The glands of Montgomery may stand out as tubercles, especially in pregnancy.

1 The examination starts with inspection, which always precedes palpation. The subject is undressed to the waist and sits upright on the side of the couch, with the examiner observing from the front. Look for lumps in the breasts and axillae, flattening of breast contour and skin dimpling.

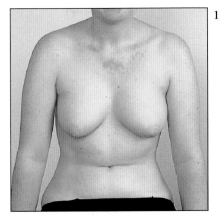

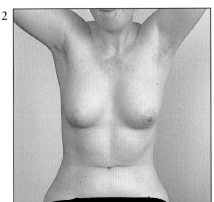

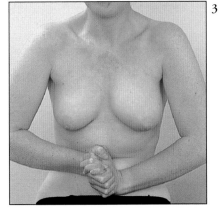

2 and 3 These features may be accentuated during arm movements and fixation. The subject's hands at first rest on the couch on either side. This is followed by raising the arms above the head and leaning forward, and then by pressing the hands together, or on the hips. To assess tethering to the serratus anterior muscles, the subject leans forward with outstretched hands against resistance.

During these movements the breasts should be observed for symmetry, the two sides compared and mobility of the breast on the chest wall assessed. Elevation may produce unequal ascent in the presence of underlying abnormalities; it also allows examination of the skin under the breasts. Note any redness, oedema, peau d'orange, ulceration, skin nodularity or abnormal venous patterns which may indicate associated pathology.

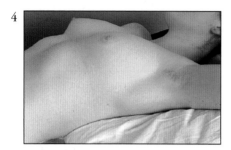

4 Palpation of the breast is undertaken with the subject lying flat on the couch with the hand on the same side placed behind the head and a pillow behind the shoulder. This position serves to relax the pectoral muscles and allow the breast to spread evenly, 'floating' on the chest wall. If an abnormality has been reported on one side, examination begins with the other: on coming to the abnormal side, ask the subject to point out the area of abnormality if it is not obvious.

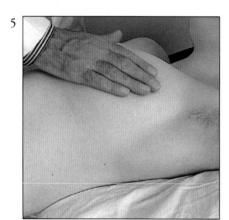

5 Palpation begins with gentle pressure and rotation of the flat of the hand over the central part of the breast.

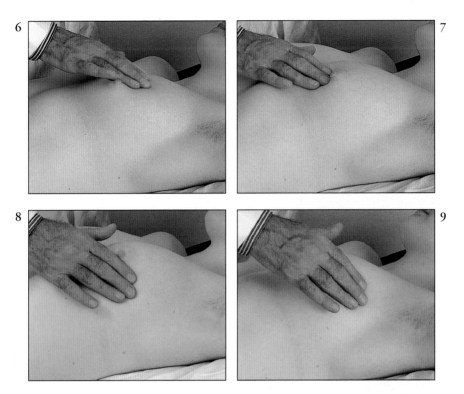

6 to 9 Examine every part of the breast systematically. A possible technique is to start with the upper inner quadrant and progress circularly to the upper outer quadrant and the axillary tail. Palpate with the flat of the outstretched fingers with rotatory and to and fro movements, gently pressing the breast tissue onto the chest wall.

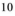

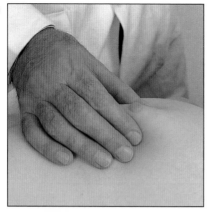

10 Be sure to gently palpate the nipple area and retroareolar tissues between finger and thumb to detect any nodularity within this region.

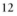

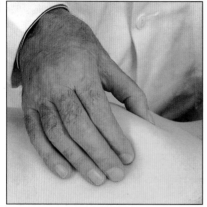

11 and 12 Abnormal areas are further palpated between finger and thumb: pendulous breasts may have to be examined bimanually. The axillary tail requires particular attention to define lumps.

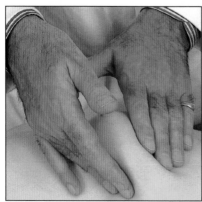

13 Note the size, shape, consistency and mobility of any abnormal areas. Tethering to underlying fascia and muscles is accentuated by asking the patient to press her hands on her hips and then moving the abnormal area to-and-fro in different directions. Superficial tethering is demonstrated by gently squeezing the overlying skin to assess whether it is free of the underlying abnormality. Normal breast tissue is commonly nodular and becomes engorged premenstrually. In doubtful cases the examination is repeated at a different time in the menstrual cycle.

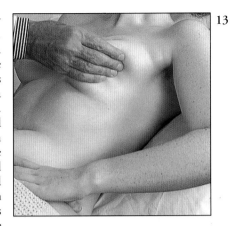

13

14 and 15 In the case of nipple discharge, particularly in galactorrhoea, gentle expression of fluid from the breast is undertaken by medio-lateral and supero-inferior expression, followed by expression from the nipple.

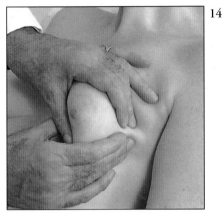

14

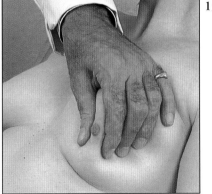

15

Axilla

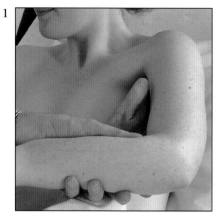 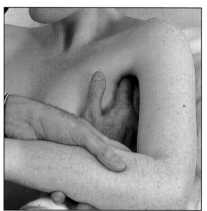

1 and 2 Examination of the axilla is a routine part of a general examination of the lymphatic system (p 48). It is of particular importance in examination of the female breast as much of the lymphatic drainage of the organ is to this group of nodes. For the left axilla, the weight of the subject's left arm is taken in the left hand of the examiner. The latter uses the right hand to first examine the anterior group of lymph nodes against the muscles and the fascia of the anterior wall of the axilla and between the pectoralis major and minor muscles.

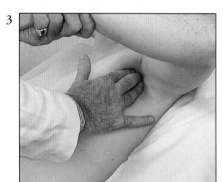 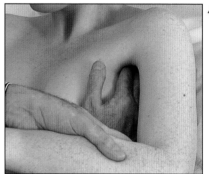

3 and 4 The cupped fingers are pressed upwards and inwards into the apex of the axilla and drawn downwards over the medial wall, to palpate the apical and medial nodes. During this manoeuvre explain what is being done and that pressure is being applied. Watch the subject's face to ensure that it does not cause any marked discomfort.

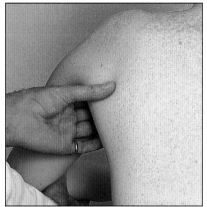
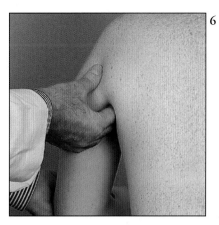

6

5 and 6 The posterior and lateral groups of axillary lymph nodes are more easily palpated from behind the subject, pressure being applied respectively to the posterior wall of the axilla, and the medial aspects of the humeral neck and shaft.

7 In examination of the right axilla the procedure is repeated, the examiner using the right hand to support the subject's right arm and palpating with the left hand. It is common to find small palpable axillary nodes in the normal subject and these are often termed 'shotty nodes'. They can be found on self-examination. Note any swelling of the arm that could be indicative of lymphatic obstruction.

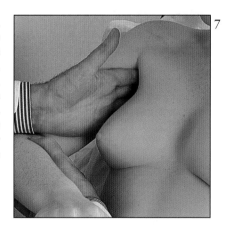

7

8
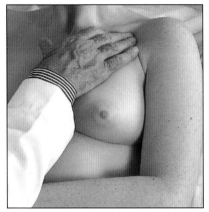
9
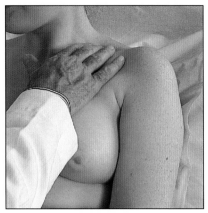

8 and 9 On completion of examination of the axilla on each side, the infraclavicular and supraclavicular fossae are palpated for their respective groups of nodes. In the latter, look particularly for the scalene node behind the lower attachment of the sternomastoid muscle (p 50).

Examination of the breast is completed by examining for hepato-megaly and tenderness along the length of the spine (pp 122, 105). Patients should also be instructed in self-examination, observing for symmetry in front of a mirror with arms at their sides, raised and pressed on hips. They should then lie with their hand behind the head and the shoulder supported on a pillow as already described, palpating with the opposite hand.

Checklist for the Assessment of the Female Breast

History

Pain: cyclical/persistent

Lump: generalised/discrete; duration, change, previous history

Discharge: milk, pus, blood, serous (colour)

Menstrual history; pregnancy; breast feeding; pill and hormone replacement

Family history

Examination

Secluded, warm area with subject undressed to waist

Sitting, reaching up, leaning forward, lying

64

For each breast: pillow behind shoulder and hand behind head

Inspection

Symmetry, mobility, flattening, swelling, skin dimpling, redness, peau d'orange, ulceration, submammary eczema, lumps

Nipple: shape, symmetry, inversion, colour, eczema, encrustation, discharge

Palpation

Examine each quadrant, the retroareolar area and the nipple for nodularity (general/focal), lumps, mobility

Express from the nipple

Axillary nodes: anterior, apical, medial, posterior, lateral, infraclavicular, supraclavicular

Liver enlargement; spinal tenderness

The Thorax

The thoracic cage is made up of the twelve thoracic vertebrae, the associated ribs and the sternum (pp 92 and 93). Anteriorly the thorax extends from the clavicles to the costal margin, which is made up of the seventh to the tenth ribs, the upper seven ribs articulating with the sternum. The second costal cartilages articulate at the sternal angle. This is a convenient point from which to count ribs and their interspaces. This is more difficult in the female, on account of the breasts, and is also a problem with generalised obesity.

The sternum can be felt from the suprasternal notch to the xiphisternum and is variable in size and shape. In the male the nipples lie approximately in the fourth intercostal space and the liver rises to this level underneath the central dome on the right side of the diaphragm.

Posteriorly, the thorax merges with the neck and lumbar regions. The vertebra prominens (C7) and the spine of the first thoracic vertebra are easily palpable, the remaining thoracic spines lie subcutaneously. The upper ribs are covered by the powerful muscles of the shoulder girdles. The scapulae overlie the second to the seventh ribs. The eleventh and twelfth ribs are usually palpable inferiorly; they overlie the kidneys. On the left side the tenth rib overlies the longitudinal axis of the spleen. With the arms abducted to 180 degrees, the lower medial border of the scapula approximates to the line of the oblique fissure of each lung.

The Cardiovascular System

The heart is subject to a wide variety of congenital defects, some of which are incompatible with life. Those encountered in clinical practice include atrial and ventricular septal defects, patent ductus arteriosus, various components of Fallot's tetralogy and coarctation of the aorta. These conditions give rise to characteristic changes of heart sounds with additional sounds, murmurs and alteration in rhythm. They may produce cardiac failure with the symptoms of dyspnoea, palpitations and peripheral oedema. In some cardiac abnormalities there is a mixing of venous and arterial blood producing cyanosis.

The cardiac valves may be congenitally abnormal or damaged after rheumatic fever. These abnormalities may be detected on clinical examination as well as by tests of cardiac function. Arteriosclerosis produces arterial stenosis and occlusion. In the coronary and cerebral vessels this gives rise to myocardial infarction and stroke respectively, and these effects are currently the commonest cause of death in the western world. Damage to the myocardium can give rise to angina (cardiac pain on exercise), abnormal cardiac rhythms and heart failure. Reduction of blood flow in the lower limbs gives rise to claudication (calf pain on exercise) and, in more severe cases, rest pain and gangrene of the feet.

In this section, the cardiac and vascular systems are considered separately. In clinical practice, it is usual to examine both the heart and the lungs from the front, before sitting a patient up to examine the back of their chest. Both cardiovascular and respiratory systems include an initial general examination, as considered on p 30. Additional points are included below. Examination of the pulses is usually undertaken regionally but in patients with arterial disease, a more systematic approach is required and this approach is taken in this chapter.

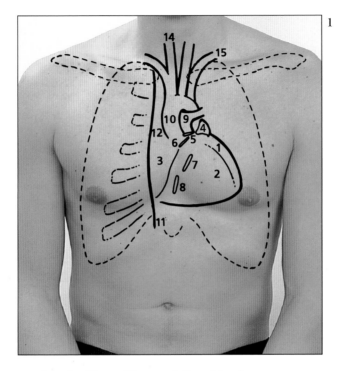

1

1 Anterior Thorax/Heart and Great Vessel

1	Left ventricle	**9**	Pulmonary trunk
2	Right ventricle	**10**	Ascending aorta
3	Right atrium	**11**	Inferior vena cava
4	Left auricular appendage	**12**	Superior vena cava
5	Pulmonary valve	**13**	Left innominate vein
6	Aortic valve	**14**	Right common carotid
7	Mitral valve		artery
8	Tricuspid valve	**15**	Left subclavian artery

The examination of the cardiovascular system begins with a general examination of the patient (p 30). Note in particular any cyanosis of the mucous membrane and any clubbing of the fingers or toes. examine the extensor tendons of the hands and later the Achilles tendon for xanthoma (indicating hyperlipidaemia).

The Pulse

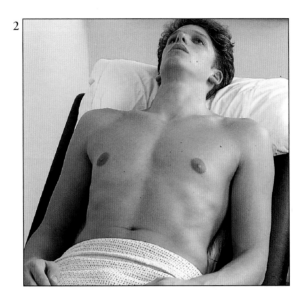

2 The examiner should first ensure the patient is lying comfortably in a semi-recumbent position at 45 degrees, with the upper half of the body exposed. In the female patient, cover the breast with a towel or loose garment. The respiratory rate should be noted, the normal resting rate being between 12 and 16 breaths per minute. Patients in heart failure are likely to have tachypnoea (increased respiration rate) with often shallow, rapid breathing exceeding 20 breaths per minute. The presence of reduced cardiac output will lead to stagnant hypoxia with evidence of peripheral and possibly central cyanosis. This can be gleaned from inspection of the hands, lips and (central cyanosis) the tongue. Abnormalities of respiration are further considered on p 92.

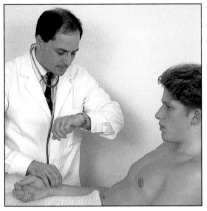

3 Next examine the hands and pulse. In the former look for evidence of clubbing and any stigmata of infective endocarditis (splinter haemorrhages, Osler's nodes). The features that should be noted in the pulse, are the rate, the volume, the character, the rhythm and the vessel wall. The rate is between 60 and 80 in fit individuals. In healthy young subjects the rate varies with the respiratory cycle. During inspiration, there is a decrease in sympathetic tone leading to cardiac acceleration. This phenomenon is known as sinus arrhythmia; it becomes less noticeable with age.

A low volume pulse may indicate low stroke volume. A bounding pulse on the other hand suggests a large pulse pressure as may be seen in a number of pathologies such a thyrotoxicosis and chronic respiratory failure. In health, the beat to beat variation in volume is virtually non-existent.

The rhythm in health will be sinus rhythm. Sinus arrhythmia as previously mentioned is a normal phenomenon. Irregular rhythms may be caused by the presence of atrial fibrillation (irregularly irregular pulse, usually obvious when the pulse is rapid), or may be caused by the presence of atrial premature beats or ventricular premature beats. With ventricular premature beats, there is usually a compensatory pause immediately after the premature beat, and the very next beat is likely to generate a larger injection volume with the larger pulse volume at the wrist.

4

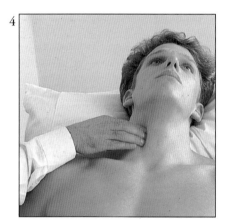

4 The character of the pulse is best determined by examining the carotid pulse. This enables a more careful analysis of the wave form. A slow rising pulse suggests aortic outflow obstruction due to either aortic stenosis or subvalvular aortic stenosis. In contrast a collapsing pulse, characterised by a rapid up and down stroke, may occur when there is significant aortic regurgitation, a patent ductus arteriosus, or arteriovenous malformations.

The anacrotic pulse (due to slow ejection of blood from the left ventricle in aortic stenosis) can be combined with a collapsing pulse to form the bisferiens pulse, which in clinical practice is difficult to elicit.

In pulsus paradoxus, deep inspiration provokes significant lowering of the pulse volume and this may occur with constrictive pericarditis, pericardial tamponade, and severe asthma. In the latter, it is caused by abnormal movement of the septum occluding the cavity of the left ventricle during systole.

The vessel wall is more easily palpable when involved in atheromatous disease.

5 The next part of the examination involves an assessment of the jugular venous pulse. The assessment of the internal jugular vein should take into consideration its surface marking (p 37). A line joining the depression between the sternal and clavicular heads of the sterno-mastoid muscle drawn, to just behind the angle of the jaw, delineates the position of the internal jugular vein. The patient, should be semi-recumbent at an angle of 45 degrees, and should have his/her head turned slightly away from the mid-line. The observer tries to detect a pulsatile movement just deep to the sternomastoid muscle. In health, the pulsation is barely visible with a patient in this position. In heart failure or pericardial constriction, the jugular venous pulse is elevated.

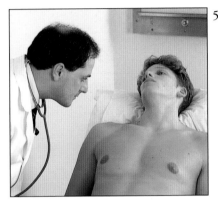

5

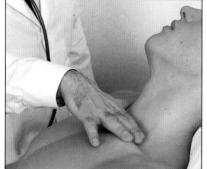

6 Occasionally it may be difficult to distinguish between a venous pulsation and an arterial pulsation in the base of the neck. Applying mild pressure to the base of the neck overlying the proximal part of the internal jugular vein will break the column of blood between the right side of the heart and the internal vein, and will obliterate venous pulsation. Such light pressure will not affect arterial pulsation.

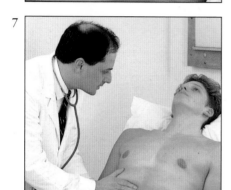

7 Another method of deciding whether a pulsation is venous or arterial is to apply light pressure over the liver which will expel more blood into the right side of the heart. If the jugular venous pulse is raised, it will rise even further with this additional venous return. The level of the jugular venous pulse will therefore rise. A non-pulsatile elevation of venous pressure is suggestive of superior vena caval obstruction.

In practice it takes a hawkish eye to pick up the composition of the jugular venous pulse and, contrary to what most textbooks say, it is virtually impossible to pick up the ACXVY components. However, whenever there is abnormality of the venous pulse, an attempt should be made to synchronise it with the arterial pulse by compressing the contralateral carotid pulse. In this way, systolic waves may be observed, indicative of tricuspid regurgitation and the occasional cannon wave, which is typical of complete heart block. Occasionally flutter waves may be seen and, if there is a 2:1 block, the venous wave will move twice as fast as the carotid rate.

This may be an appropriate moment to record the blood pressure (p 36). This should be undertaken at a set point in the cardiovascular or general examination, so that this important measurement is not ommitted. If different volume radial pulses exist, blood pressure is measured in both arms. In patients with elevated blood pressures, or those being treated for hypertension, it may be appropriate to measure standing and lying blood pressures.

Examination of the Precordium

Examination of the thorax can be subdivided into inspection, palpation, percussion and auscultation. Cardiac percussion is considered with the respiratory system where this sub-division is more complete.

In health, depending on the thickness of the thoracic wall, the apex beat, that is the lower and most outer point at which the cardiac pulse may be felt, may be visible. With thicker chest walls this is not so. Abnormal shape of the precordium should be noted together with any scars. Asymmetry of the parasternal costal areas may be indicative of underlying right ventricular or left ventricular hypertrophy.

8 The normal apex is located around the 5th intercostal space, in the mid-clavicular line. In order to locate it, the whole hand should be applied to the area just below the nipple in both males and females. In the female, the examiner will have to lift the breast in order to observe and palpate the appropriate area; a mitral valvotomy scar is easily missed if this observation is not made. The costal cartiliages are counted down from the second, this being opposite the sternal angle.

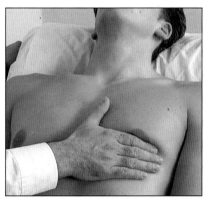

Displacement of the apex beat may be due to movement of the mediastinum or true cardiac enlargement. The left ventricle normally produces the apex beat and, when the ventricle is hypertrophied, the beat is forceful and may extend outwards towards the axilla. This hyperdynamic pulse of left ventricular hypertrophy, is in contrast to the hyperkinetic and rather sustained impulse characteristic of volume overload of the ventricle. The latter may occur in heart failure, and mitral and aortic regurgitation. Palpation of the precordium may reveal an abnormal pulsation due for example to an aneurysm of the left ventricle.

A tapping effect is highly suggestive of mitral stenosis. Occasionally, a dyskinetic impulse may be due to transmission of a powerful atrial contraction (causing a fourth sound) and this typically occurs in hypertrophic obstructive cardiomyopathy (HOCM) and in systemic hypertension. A dyskinetic impulse may also result from a left ventricular aneurysm.

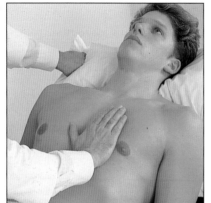

9 When the hand is placed firmly over the precordium just lateral to the sternum on the left, abnormal impulses from the right ventricle may be felt, as for example in right ventricular hypertrophy due to pulmonary hypertension. This is felt with the base of the hand.

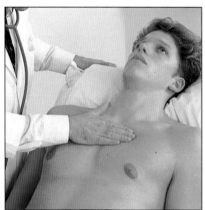

10 If the pulmonary artery is dilated and palpable, it is felt in the 2nd left intercostal space during expiration.

Other pulsations may be observed. An arterial impulse in the suprasternal notch may indicate an unfolded aorta and abnormal arterial pulses in the neck may result from the tortuosity and hardening of the carotid arteries. In thin patients, especially if affected by chronic airways obstruction, it is not unusual for a pulsation to be detected in the epigastrium.

Thrills indicate turbulent flow usually through a small orifice such as a narrowed valve or a ventricular septal defect. They are usually systolic, i.e. a thrill which coincides in time with the apex beat, but may also occur in diastole.

11 The presence of a thrill almost always indicates an organic lesion. In order to detect a thrill, it may be necessary to lean the patient forward during expiration and apply the palm of the hand to the base of the heart. The pulmonary component of the second sound may also be palpable. In this position also palpate for thrills over the apex.

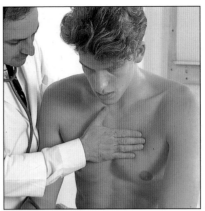

Auscultation of the Heart

The examiner should note at each site the quality of the first and second heart sounds, and whether there are any additional sounds. The first heart sound has two components, caused by mitral and tricuspid valve closure. Mitral closure occurs slightly before tricuspid but this does not normally cause splitting of the sound. The second heart sound is at a slightly lower pitch than the first and occurs at the end of systole. It comprises both aortic and pulmonary valve closure. A useful mnemonic is that these valves close in alphabetical order, i.e. aortic before pulmonary.

During inspiration, splitting of the second sound may be found over the pulmonary area, this being caused by the increased venous return to the right ventricle, leading to more prolonged systole on the right side of the heart.

Splitting of the first heart sound may indicate complete right bundle branch block whereas increase of the normal splitting of the second heart sound will occur if there is delay in right ventricular emptying, as might occur in right bundle branch block, pulmonary stenosis, ventricular septal defects, and mitral incompetence.

Atrial septal defects typically cause a fixed splitting of the second sound. Reverse splitting of the second sound (i.e. splitting occuring in expiration, as opposed to inspiration) is normally ascribed to delayed left ventricle depolarization (e.g. left bundle branch block) and delayed left ventricular emptying (e.g. aortic stenosis, coarctation of the aorta, patent ductus arterosis).

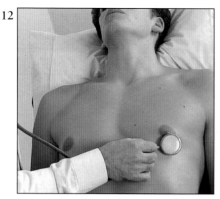 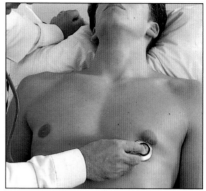

12 The examination starts in the mitral area with the bell of the stethoscope. This produces a resonating chamber that is particularly efficient in amplifying low pitched sounds such as might occur with mitral diastolic murmurs or a fourth heart sound. The bell is applied lightly to the chest wall at the apex.

13 Next, the diaphragm is used and this is appropriate for the detection of high pitched sounds such as those generated by systolic murmurs.

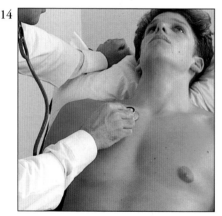 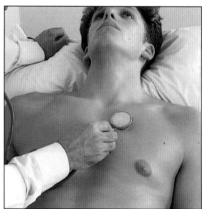

14 to 16 The stethoscope is then placed systematically over the aortic area (2nd right intercostal space), the pulmonary area (2nd left intercostal space) and finally the tricuspid areas (5th left intercostal space). At each site both the bell and the diaphragm are used for auscultation.

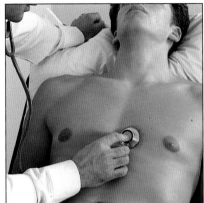

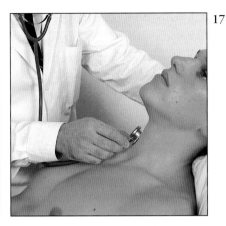

17 The above order of auscultation links the mitral and aortic valves and the pulmonary with the tricuspid, i.e. the valves of the respective sides of the heart. Auscultation must not be limited to these four sites. When abnormalities are found or suspected (see below), the stethoscope is moved over each area to identify positions of optimal sound and also to follow the radiation of sound, typical sites being along the left sternal border and radiation into the left axilla and into the right side of the neck.

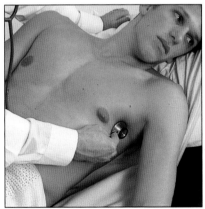

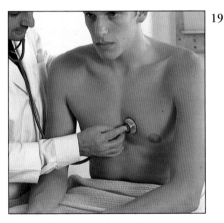

19

18 and 19 Repositioning a patient may also accentuate sounds, such as turning to the left lateral position or sitting upright, and sounds may further be accentuated by deep inspiration or deep expiration or a Valsalva manoeuvre.

Additional Heart Sounds

The third heart sound is a low pitched diastolic sound usually best heard over the apex. It is probably caused by tautening of the mitral and tricuspid capillary muscles at the end of rapid diastolic filling. It usually indicates left ventricular dysfunction.

A fourth heart sound is a late diastolic sound, slightly more high pitched than the third. It is never physiological, and usually reflects poor ventricular compliance (e.g. aortic stenosis, systemic hypertension, HOCM).

Extra Sounds Within the Heart

Murmurs: Added sounds, such as murmurs should be assessed systematically and associated peripheral signs sought. The timing of the murmur (i.e. systolic or diastolic), the area of greatest intensity, its loudness and the effect of various manoeuvres, such as inspiration and a Valsalva, are all required to maximise the information on a likely underlying cause.

Systolic murmurs can be pansystolic, ejection systolic or late systolic. Pansystolic murmurs extend throughout systole beginning with the first heart sound and going right up to the second heart sound. The loudness of pitch may vary during systole and common causes include mitral regurgitation. The intensity of mid-systolic murmurs (or ejection murmurs) is greatest in mid-systole. The usual cause is turbulent fluid through a narrowed aortic or pulmonary valve. Late systolic murmurs typically occur in conditions such as mitral valve prolapse or capillary muscle dysfunction.

Diastolic murmurs may be either early, where they usually have a deep crescendo quality (e.g. caused by pulmonary or aortic regurgitation), or mid-diastolic. The latter, begin later in diastole, are usually short, extending up to the first sound: they have a low pitched quality. Their usual cause is impairment of blood flow in ventricular filling, such as caused by mitral or tricuspid stenosis. Pre-systolic murmurs are caused by atrial systole across a narrow valve. Continuous murmurs may be caused by a patent ductus arteriosus, arteriovenous shunts and congenital aorto-pulmonary windows. Rarer causes include a ruptured sinus of Valsalva and a coronary artery fistula.

The area of intensity of a murmur is important. For example, mitral regurgitation is best heard at the apex and radiates towards the axilla while others may be heard over the entire precordium. Conduction of an injection systolic murmur into the carotid artery suggests an aortic valvular origin of the lesion. Loudness of atrial murmurs is not clinically relevant and, paradoxically, more severe lesions may produce quieter murmurs.

Dynamic manoeuvres, such as inspiration, should be employed to evaluate murmurs. Inspiration increases venous return and therefore blood flow through the right side of the heart, usually accentuating right sided murmurs.

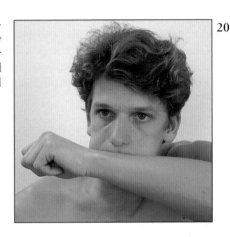

20 A Valsalva manoeuvre is performed by asking the patient to blow hard on the back of his/her hand or forearm without releasing air. It will change the murmurs of HOCM and mitral valve prolapse.

A pericardial friction rub may be audible over the base of the heart with the patient leaning forward; it is caused by the movement of inflamed pericardial surfaces rubbing against each other.

The cardiac examination is completed by listening over the base of the lungs for evidence of crepitations caused by pulmonary oedema (p 101).

If the clinical features suggest tricuspid regurgitation, an attempt should be made to elicit pulsatility of the liver. This is best done during deep inspiration with the patient supine and the examiner's hands sandwiching the liver, accentuating the abnormal pulsation (p 72). This is an extremely useful sign, together with the systolic waves in the jugular venous pulse of tricuspid regurgitation. Note that ascites may result from severe right heart failure.

Cardiac Murmurs

Cardiac murmurs can be classified by their timing, position, pitch and grade. Figure **21** illustrates the relation of commonly heard murmurs to the heart sounds and ventricular systoli and diastoli. Subsequent figures indicate the combination of heart sounds and murmurs that are typical of some common disorders.

The site of maximum intensity and any radiation provides information on the underlying disease. High pitched sounds are best heard with the bell of the stethoscope and low pitched sounds with the diaphragm. Grades are from I to VI. I: very soft. II: soft but easily audible. III: moderately loud. IV: loud with associated thrill. V: very loud plus thrill. VI: maximum loudness with thrill, heard without a stethoscope.

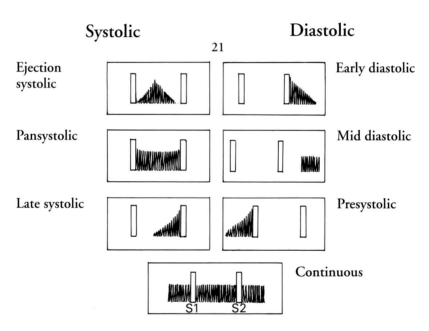

S_1, S_2: first and second heart sounds

Mitral stenosis:

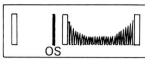

Low-pitched diastolic rumble, with presystolic accentuation if no AF, localised to the apex, Loud S_1 and opening snap (OS).

Mitral regurgitation:

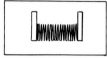

Blowing or musical pansystolic murmur, merging into soft second sound.

Mitral valve prolapse:

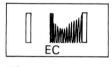

Murmur follows midsystolic ejection click (EC), with late systolic accentuation, heard best at apex.

Aortic stenosis:

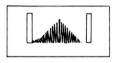

Systolic ejection murmur, aortic area radiating to neck, soft second sound.

Aortic regurgitation:

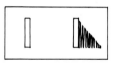

High-pitched early diastolic murmur, left sternal edge, maximum when leaning forward in full expiration.

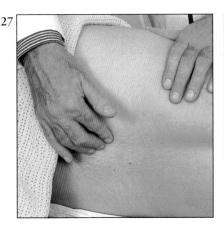
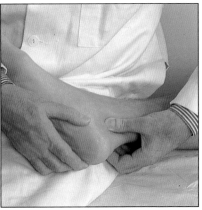

27 and 28   Pitting oedema is best sought below the knee or in the sacral area. When extensive, it may involve the thighs and creep up the anterior abdominal wall. The hallmark is pitting, which occurs when applying light pressure to the skin. This can be demonstrated by pressure in front of the Achilles tendons or over the shins. The latter may cause discomfort so watch the patient's face.

Examination of the Pulses

The remainder of the cardiovascular examination requires the systematic palpation and auscultation of peripheral pulses.

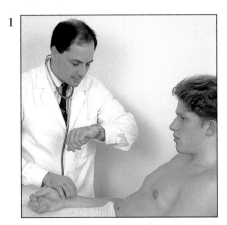

1   To feel a pulse effectively it is compressed on a firm adjacent structure, usually a bone. The distal of three fingers is used to compress the vessel while the proximal two assess the rate, rhythm, volume and character of the pulse: rolling the vessel indicates normal or thickened vessel wall. Commence by examining the radial pulses at the wrist, compressing the vessels on the lower end of each radius.

2 Radial and femoral pulses are compared for radio-femoral delay, as seen in coarctation of the aorta.

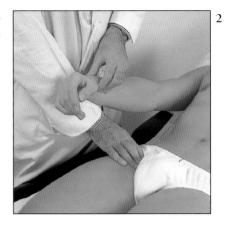

2

3 It is useful to compare the two sides of the body and also to compare the apical rate with an upper limb or cervical pulse to look for missed beats as for instance in atrial fibrillation.

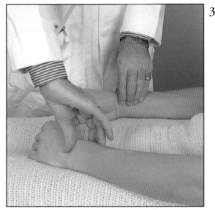

3

4 The ulnar artery passes superficial to the lateral aspect of the flexor retinaculum and is very prominent in some individuals.

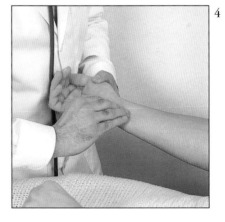

4

5 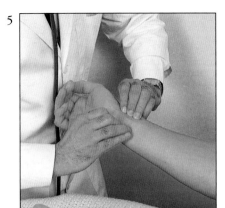 If the fist is clenched firmly, the radial and ulnar arteries are both compressed, when the fist is released return of capillary circulation is slow. The relative contribution of these two vessels to the circulation of the hand can be assessed by the effect of individual compression.

6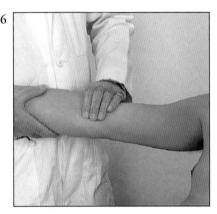

6 and 7 The brachial artery lies superficial at the level of the elbow joint, although partly covered by the bicipital aponeurosis. To facilitate palpation the elbow is fully extended to allow compression against the lower end of the humerus. It is at this site that the pulse is usually auscultated when measuring the blood pressure. The brachial artery can also be palpated against the mid-shaft of the humerus, in the grove between brachialis and biceps muscles. The axillary artery can be palpated against the head of the humerus by deep, lateral palpation in the depths of the axilla.

7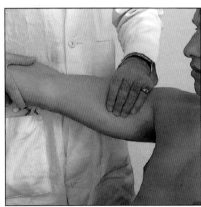

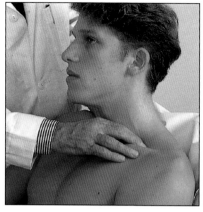

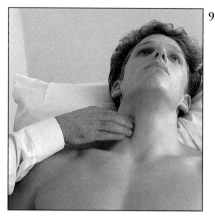

8 The subclavian artery can be palpated by compression against the first rib. This is in the posterior triangle of the neck just behind the middle of the clavicle.

9 The common carotid arteries can be palpated in the mid-cervical region, pressing backwards on the transverse processes of the cervical vertebrae.

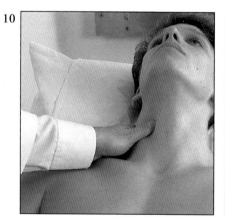

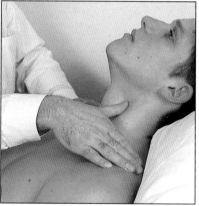

10 and 11 Unilateral or bilateral carotid compression is undertaken in this region. The common carotid bifurcation can be felt more distally towards the angle of the mandible; the external and internal branches are difficult to define independently.

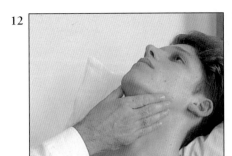
12

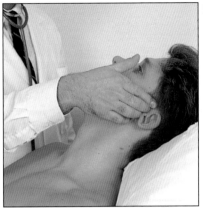
13

12 Palpate the facial artery on the inferior margin of the mandible, just anterior to the masseter muscle. The border of the muscle can be identified by asking the subject to clench his teeth.

13 Palpate the superficial temporal artery at a preauricular level or its anterior division as it crosses the temple.

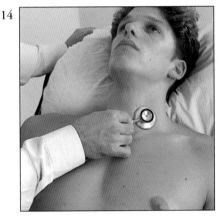
14

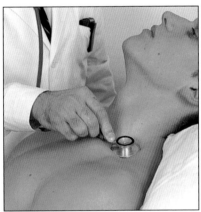
15

14 and 15 Listen to the carotid arteries in the mid-cervical region and over the carotid bifurcation, the subclavian over the first rib, the aorta at the level of the umbilicus, the iliac vessels from the aortic bifurcation to the mid-inguinal points (p 128) and the femoral arteries beyond this level. The superficial femoral and popliteal arteries are auscultated at the level of the adductor canal and over the popliteal fossa.

16 Soft bruits are commonly found over major arteries, even in normal individuals. However, stenotic disease often produces high pitched and prominent sounds. These, together with other symptoms and signs of ischaemia, prompt the observer to progress to more detailed investigation of the vascular tree.

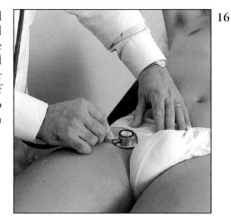

16

17 The femoral arteries are palpated over the midinguinal points, compressing each artery backwards onto the head of the femur. The two sides are compared for volume; this may be different in lower limb vascular disease.

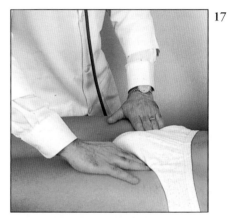

17

18 The popliteal artery is palpated against the upper end of the tibia, the knee being slightly flexed and the muscles relaxed. The pulps of all eight fingers are used to compress the artery on the tibia between the heads of gastrocnemius.

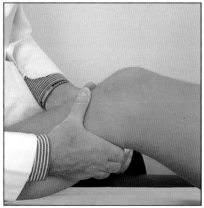

18

19

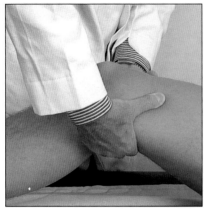

20

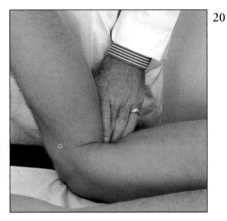

19 and 20 The popliteal artery is deeply situated in the popliteal fossa, but can be palpated against the lower end of the femur with the patient supine or prone. This is particularly useful if the distal popliteal artery is occluded.

21

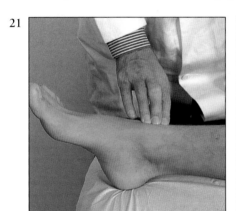

22

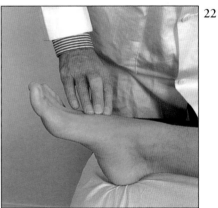

21 and 22 The anterior tibial artery crosses the ankle joint midway between the two malleoli, becoming the dorsalis pedis at this point. It then passes towards the first interdigital web. It is palpated over the heads of the metatarsals just lateral to the extensor hallucis longus tendon.

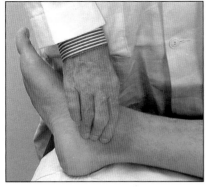 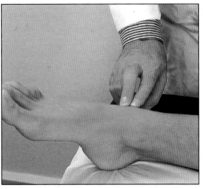

23 The posterior tibial artery passes into the foot. It can be palpated over the talus, midway between the medial malleolus and the medial prominence of the heel.

24 An anterior perforating branch from the peroneal artery can be palpated just in front of the lateral malleolus. The vessel may be palpable in the normal individual or may become prominent with occlusion of other foot vessels.

Foot pulses can be difficult to feel and the examiner can be confused by feeling the pulsation in the examining fingers. If in doubt, palpate an easily palpable wrist or femoral pulse at the same time, or count out the beats of the palpated pulse while a second observer compares this with the pulse rate taken at another prominent site.

25 In severe ischaemia the blood pressure at the ankle is markedly reduced and, as this approaches zero, elevation of the foot will produce blanching and venous emptying. In extreme cases, a gutter replaces the line of the vein.

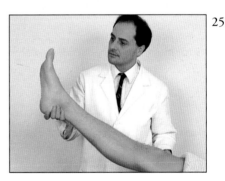 **25**

On dropping the legs over the side of the bed, in an ischaemic limb, the veins fill over a number of seconds and there is reactive hyperaemia in the feet after 1 to 3 minutes. In cases of severe ischaemia there may also be trophic changes in the toes. Examine between each pair of toes for ulceration, and the lateral side of the foot and the heel for evidence of fissuring or infection.

Checklist for the Assessment of the Cardiovascular System

History

Pain: angina; central chest (radiation); back

Palpitations; oedema; cyanosis; fatigue; syncope

Cough, sputum, haemoptysis; dyspnoea, orthopnea, paroxysmal nocturnal dyspnoea

Hypertension; diabetes; hypercholesterolaemia; smoking; family history of vascular disease

Symptoms of stroke

Claudication; pain in feet at rest; foot ulceration; gangrene

Examination

General
Marfan's, Down's, Turner's syndromes, cachexia

Hands, fingers and nails: clubbing; peripheral cyanosis; nicotine staining; splinter haemorrhages; Osler's nodes

Head and neck: jugular venous pressure (cannon waves, CV systolic waves); hepatojugular reflux; xanthelasma; pallor; jaundice; central cyanosis; malar flush; fundi

Arterial pulse: rate, rhythm, volume, character, thickening of vessel wall; tachycardia, bradycardia, sinus arrhythmia; premature beats; atrial fibrillation, hyperdynamic; collapsing (Corrigan), Bisferiens alternans; pulsus paradoxus

Radio-femoral delay; radial asyncrony; radial asymmetry

Peripheral pulses: presence, symmetry, volume, bruits

Blood pressure: Korotkoff sounds I, IV, V (appearance, muffling, disappearance), standing/lying

Respiratory rate; temperature

Heart
Examination carried out initially lying at 45 degrees; repeated in supine, rotated and sitting positions, and after Valsalva and squatting manoeuvres, to accentuate focal abnormal signs

Inspection, palpation, percussion

Scars; position, force and character of apex beat; abnormal pulsation; thrills; cardiac outline

Auscultation

Undertaken with bell and diaphragm over mitral, aortic, pulmonary and tricuspid areas: repeat during inspiration and expiration, and in various positions, as appropriate

Sounds
First and second, splitting; third and fourth, summation gallop; opening snap, ejection click, mid/late systolic click; pericardial knock/rub

Murmurs
Timing of onset and offset in relation to systoli, diastoli and valve closure

Character; point of maximum intensity; grade; radiation; effect of positional and respiratory manoeuvres

Systolic: aortic stenosis, HOCM, mitral regurgitation, mitral valve prolapse; ventricular septal defect

Diastolic: aortic regurgitation, mitral stenosis

Continuous: patent ductus arteriosus; venous hum, pulmonary arterio-venous malformation, ruptured coronary sinus

Lungs
Particularly examine for basal crepitations

Hepatomegaly, liver pulsation; pulmonary effusions; ascites; peripheral oedema

Feet
Trophic changes, pressure sores, ulceration, gangrene, inflammation, abscess formation, neuropathy, postural changes, venous filling time

The Respiratory System

Pulmonary diseases present with dyspnoea, cough, cyanosis and chest pain, and the signs of cardiac failure. Common chest diseases encountered are asthma, chronic bronchitis, emphysema, pneumonia and carcinoma of the bronchus. The latter produces local respiratory problems and its metastases may also produce associated symptoms in the bone, brain and liver. The sputum should be examined for colour, volume and consistency, noting in particular the presence of blood.

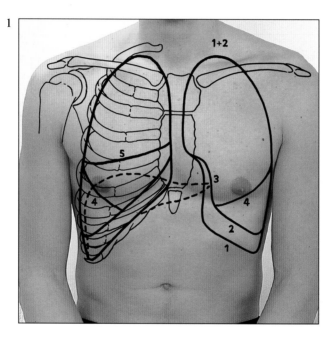

1   Anterior Thorax/Pleura and Lungs

   1   Pleural markings
   2   Lung markings
   3   Cardiac notch of left lung
   4   Oblique fissures
   5   Horizontal fissure

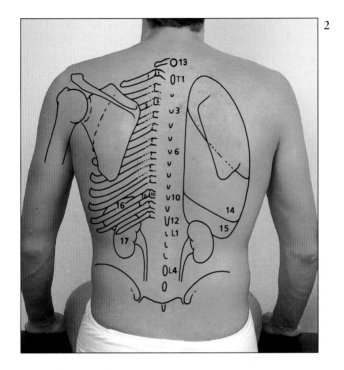

2 Posterior Aspect of the Thorax

1 to 12 Spines, transverse processes and ribs (as numbered)
13   Spine and transverse process of 7th cervical vertebra (note the down-ward direction of the transverse process compared with the upward direc-tion of T1)
14   Lower limit of right lung
15   Lower limit of pleural cavity
16   Spleen
17   Kidney and renal pelvis

Inspection

The patient should be undressed to the waist—in the case of a female, explain the need to expose the front of the chest to examine the heart and lungs. A patient may be lying semirecumbant or, ideally, should be seated with feet hanging over the side of the bed. The examiner stands back and observes the patient for evidence of dyspnoea (difficulty with respiration), tachypnoea (count the respiratory rate), the use of accessory muscles of respiration, intercostal indrawing of the lower ribs, cyanosis and any evidence of cachexia.

The back (at this stage if sitting up or later when the posterior aspect of the chest is examined) should be inspected for evidence of scoliosis or kyphosis or any other deformities, such as thoracotomy scars and prominent veins. Common deformities of the anterior chest wall include pectus excavatum (indrawn sternum) and pectus carinatum (pigeon chest).

3 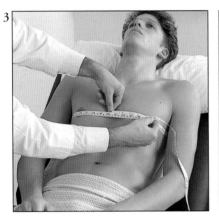 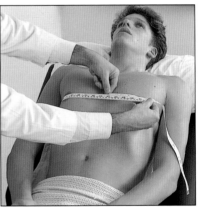 4

3 and 4 Note the position of the nipples, and whether the thoracic cavity is expanded, such as in the barrel chest of emphysema. The chest expansion is measured from inspiration to expiration, using a tape measure.

Several types of abnormal breathing patterns may be discerned at the bedside. In Cheyne-Stokes breathing, periods of apnoea (cessation of respiratory movements) alternate with periods of hyperpnoea (deep inspirations). This is due to a delay in the medullary chemoreceptor response to blood gas changes, and can occur in left ventricular failure, brain damage, chronic hypoxaemia and at high altitudes.

In Kussmaul breathing (air hunger), there is deep, rapid respiration due to stimulation of the respiratory centre. This typically occurs in diabetic ketoacidosis and lactic acidosis. Ataxic breathing (irregular in timing and depth) occurs in brainstem damage.

The examiner should listen carefully for abnormalities in breathing, such as noise, wheezing and coughing. Stridor is a continuous rasping or croaking noise causing obstruction to the larynx, and accentuated in inspiration. It may signify the presence of a foreign body, tumour or inflammatory process in the trachea. The voice should be listened to. Hoarseness may signify a recurrent laryngeal nerve palsy.

Next, pick up the hands, noting clubbing and evidence of peripheral cyanosis, nicotine staining and anaemia. Wasting of the muscles of the hand may signify a first thoracic nerve lesion, such as caused by a superior sulcus tumour. The wrist should be palpated for tenderness (caused by symmetrical periostitis of hypertrophic pulmonary osteoarthropathy) and the radial pulse inspected for pulsus paradoxus (p 71). Look at the face, observing the pupils for evidence of Horner's syndrome (p 148), anaemia within the conjunctivae and central cyanosis (tip of the tongue).

The sputum should be examined as a matter of routine. The volume and type should be noted (purulent, mucoid or mucopurulent), a large purulent volume suggesting bronchiectasis. Pink frothy sputum occurs in pulmonary oedema. Evidence of haemoptysis (coughing blood) should be sought.

Palpation

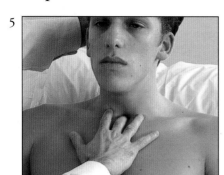

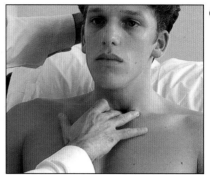

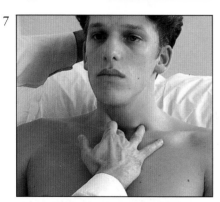

5 to 7 Note the position of the trachea in the suprasternal region. Ask the patient to relax the sternomastoid muscles by dropping his chin, and to lean slightly forward. Rest the middle finger on the suprasternal notch and pass it on either side of the trachea as deeply and inferiorly as possibly. The latter is important because even gross tracheal deviation may be missed if the examining finger comes into contact with the trachea at too high a level.

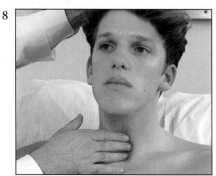

8 A tracheal tug indicates the presence of significant lung fibrosis or severe airflow obstruction. It is demonstrated when the finger resting on the trachea feels it moving inferiorly during inspiration

Ask the patient to cough, to check whether there is a loose cough, a dry cough or a bovine cough. The latter occurs when a vocal cord is paralysed and the two cannot be approximated, as in recurrent laryngeal nerve palsy (p 153). Next, ask the patient to take a maximum inspiration and blow out as rapidly and as forcefully as possible. Listen carefully, as it may be possible to discern wheeze and prolongation of the expiration phase, suggesting chronic airflow limitation. The supraclavicular fossae should be palpated for lymphadenopathy. This may be undertaken from the front, but the pulps of the fingers can be inserted deep to the clavicle more easily from behind. Supraclavicular nodes of interest in pulmonary disease include the scalene lymph nodes which are deep to the sternomastoid muscle insertion (p 50).

9
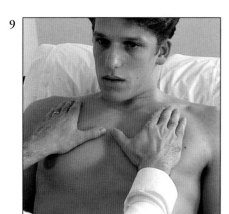

10
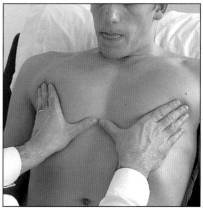

9 to 11 Expansion of the chest is tested with the palms of the hands resting symmetrically, first superiorly, then on the middle and finally on the lower chest wall with the thumbs pointing towards the midline. This is done in order to pick up possible asymmetries of expansion which are highly suggestive of underlying pulmonary disease.

11
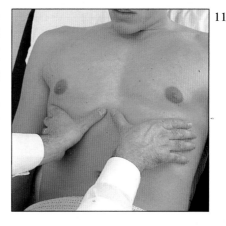

Percussion

12 to 17 Percussion requires considerable practice, and the ability to percuss well is obvious to an observer, and usually denotes that a student has spent a reasonable amount of time on the wards. Percussion of the lungs starts at the apex, bearing in mind that there are 1 or 2cm of lung above the clavicle. The clavicle is then percussed directly by the percussing finger. The rest of the lung is percussed initially anteriorly, then within the axillae. The same areas of the two sides are percussed consecutively for comparative purposes, although only one side is shown in the figures in each case.

The percussion may be either resonant, dull or stony dull. A hyper-reonant tone may indicate an underlying pneumothorax although in practice this is usually wishful thinking. The axillae are best percussed by asking the patient to raise the arms above the head, the examiner taking care to move fingers as high up in the axilla as possible. Failure to do the latter may lead to the missing of vital physical signs.

Also use coarse percussion, where 3 or 4 fingers are tapped lightly on each side and a comparison made of each (p 103). This can pick up stony dullness which is then precisely mapped by more careful percussion. On percussion posteriorly, the scapulae should be moved out of the way by asking the patient to move his elbows forward. This rotates the scapulae anteriorly.

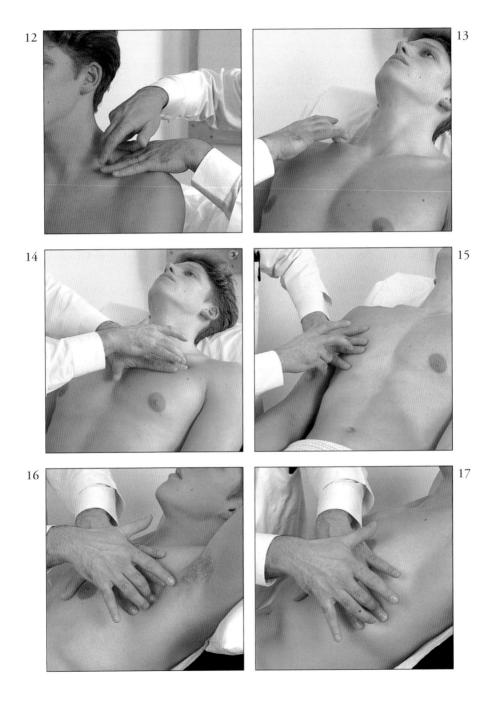

Auscultations

Normal breath sounds are produced by the airways rather than the alveoli. They have been likened to wind rustling in leaves, and are called vesicular sounds. *Vesicular sounds* are louder and longer on inspiration than expiration, there being no gap between inspiration and expiration. These sounds are generated by the turbulence of air in the large airways filtering through the normal lung to the chest wall.

Bronchial breath sounds have a more hollow and blowing nature. They are audible throughout expiration and there is often a gap between inspiration and expiration. The expiratory sound has a higher intensity than the inspiratory sound. They are normally audible over the trachea and the main bronchi, as well as over areas of consolidation.

Breath sounds should be described as normal or reduced in quality. Causes of reduced breath sounds include emphysema, pleural effusion, pneumothorax and pleural thickening.

Adventitious sounds are either wheezes (rhonchi) or crackles (râles). Wheezes have a musical quality and may be heard both in inspiration and expiration. They are caused by continuous oscillation of opposing airway walls and imply airway narrowing. The pitch depends on the speed of airway flow.

Auscultation over the chest while the patient utters some words (e.g. 'ninety nine'), vocal resonance, gives further information about the lung's ability to transmit sound. Over the normal lung, the low-pitched components of speech are heard with a booming quality and high-pitched sounds are attenuated. In consolidation, high pitched sounds are preferentially transmitted and the speech heard through the stethoscope has a bleating or aegophonous quality. When vocal resonance is increased to a great extent, even whispered speech may become audible, a sign known as whispering pectoriloquy.

An alternative method is to look for tactile vocal fremitus, the side of the examiner's hand being placed over each lung during enunciation (p 103); this is notoriously unreliable.

The figures thus far have been illustrating the examination of the anterior chest. The text however, relates to both anterior and posterior examination, and examination of the back of the chest follows the same order: inspection, palpation, percussion and auscultation, using identical techniques. Again, equivalent sites on the two sides are examined consecutively, but the illustrations only show one side at each site.

18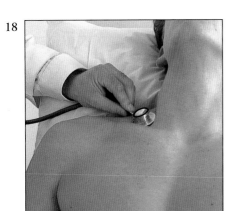

19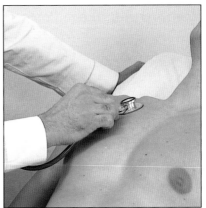

20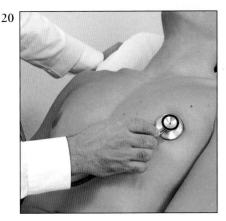

21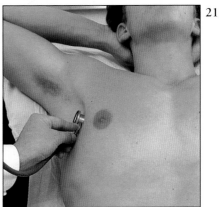

18 to 22 The chest is auscultated, first in the apices and then in the upper, mid and low zones, anteriorly within the axillae and, finally, posteriorly. Use the diaphragm of the stethoscope to assess the breath sounds. The patient is asked to take a moderately deep breath and breathe out through the mouth. Excessive inspiration and too complete an expiration may precipipitate the symptoms and signs of hypocarbia, the patient feeling faint.

22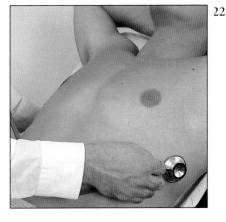

Examination of the Posterior Aspect of the Chest

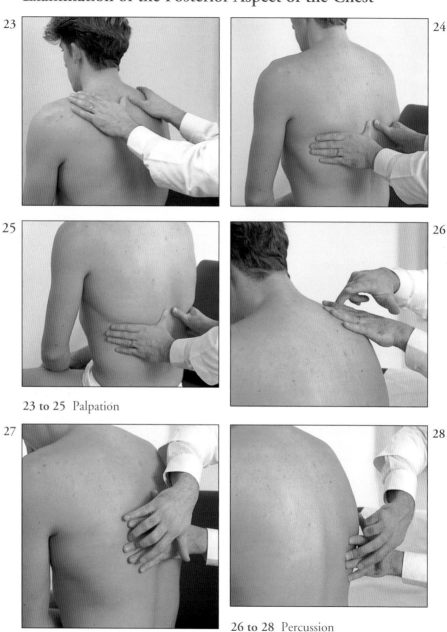

23 to 25 Palpatión

26 to 28 Percussion

29 Coarse percussion

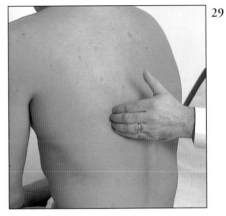

29

30

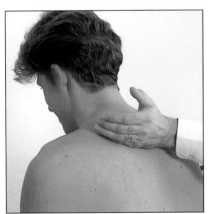

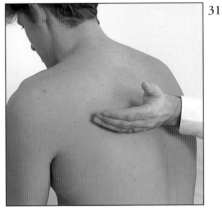

31

30 to 32 Tactile vocal fremitus

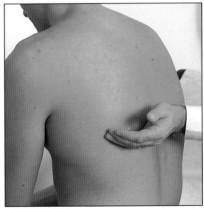

32

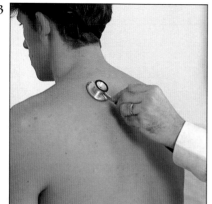

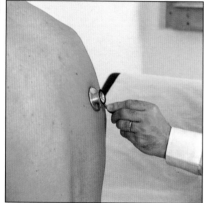

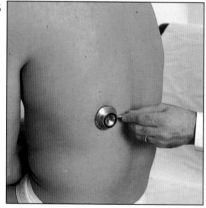

Examining for Vertebral Tenderness

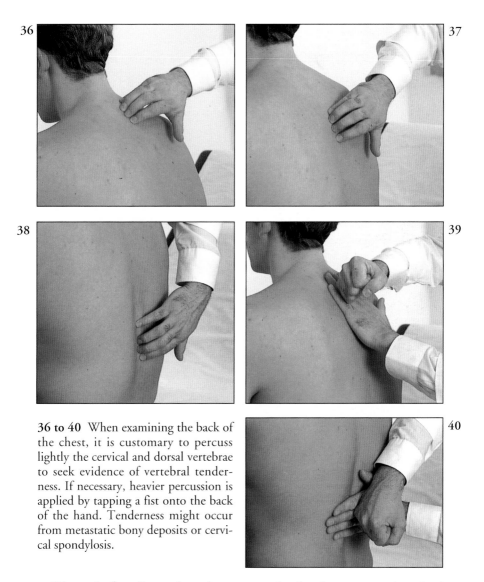

36 to 40 When examining the back of the chest, it is customary to percuss lightly the cervical and dorsal vertebrae to seek evidence of vertebral tenderness. If necessary, heavier percussion is applied by tapping a fist onto the back of the hand. Tenderness might occur from metastatic bony deposits or cervical spondylosis.

The end of cardiac and respiratory examination is an appropriate time to examine the breasts and axillae (p 56), if a patient's symptoms have not already directed the examination to these areas.

Checklist for the Assessment of the Respiratory System

History

Cough: night time, dry, productive, sputum (appearance and volume); haemoptysis

Chest pain: related to respiration; angina

Breathlessness: at rest, on exercise, orthopnoea, paroxysmal nocturnal dyspnoea; wheezing

Pyrexia; myalgia; rigors; cyanosis; oedema

Upper respiratory tract infection: nasal discharge; nasal obstruction pain over sinuses and in ears; cervical lymphadenopathy

Examination

General
Pulse; blood pressure; respiratory rate; temperature

Hands, fingers and nails: clubbing; peripheral cyanosis; nicotine staining; wasting of small muscles; wrist tenderness; carbon dioxide retention flap

Head and neck: conjunctival pallor; jugular venous pressure; Horner's syndrome; hoarseness of voice

Cervical and axillary nodes

NB: cough, sputum (examine sputum pot—colour, consistency, volume)

Chest

Inspection

Scars; prominent veins

Pattern of respiration: rate, depth, tachypnoea, dyspnoea, irregularity, stridor, use of accessory muscles, Cheyne-Stokes

Anterior chest wall configuration: pectus excavatum, pectus carinatum

Vertebral column abnormalities: buffalo hump, barrel chest, lordosis, kyphoscoliosis

Palpation

Tracheal deviation, tracheal tug

Chest expansion: tape measure and manual assessment

Tactile vocal fremitus; subcutaneous emphysema; rib tenderness

Percussion

Resonant, hyper-resonant, dull, stony dull

Coarse percussion

Auscultation—use bell and diaphragm

Breath sounds: normal, vesicular, bronchial, bronchiovesicular

Adventitious sounds: crackles (râles), wheezes (rhonchi)

Vocal resonance: aegophony, whispering pectoriliquay

Pleural friction rub

The Alimentary System

The alimentary tract starts at the mouth and extends to the anus. Thus, examination includes these areas as well as the abdomen. Disease of the alimentary tract may also produce systemic effects and alimentary examination commences with

(a) the *hands*, followed by

(b) the *mouth*,

(c) the *conjunctivae and sclera* (p 38), for subconjunctival pallor and jaundice, and

(d) the *root of the neck* (p 49), for supraclavicular lymphadenopathy.

The Hands (p 33)

In the hands, the nails may show pallor and/or koilonychia. Clubbing may be present in chronic liver and bowel disease. Liver damage may also produce palmar erythema and spider naevi.

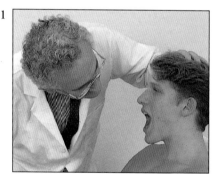

Mouth and Neck

1 Halitosis (bad breath) may be due to bad teeth, and infection and ulceration of the gums or oral mucosa. Other causes include bronchiectasis and intestinal obstruction. Ketoacidosis, uraemia and hepatic failure have specific foetors, as do alcohol and certain drugs, such as paraldehyde.

A torch, tongue depressor and disposable gloves are useful accessories for detailed inspection and palpation of the mouth when local disease is suspected. The lips may be dry and fissured, and fissuring of the angles of the mouth may accompany nutritional problems and anaemia.

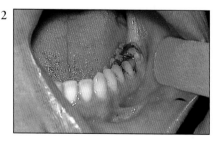

2 Note the number and the state of the teeth.

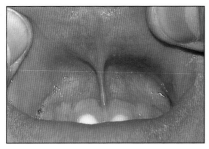

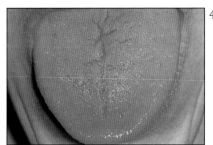

3 Normal gums are closely applied to the teeth but may recede and become infected or, in some conditions, hypertrophic. In edentulous subjects examine the gums for evidence of damage from dentures.

4 The tongue may be dehydrated, fissured or ulcerated. Various coatings and contours may be of no clinical significance but the changes of leukoplakia (white raised patches) must be recognised as premalignant.

5 A geographic tongue is a normal variant, as may be ethnic pigmentation. Note also mouth ulceration, tonsillar enlargement, fauceal or pharyngeal erythema and nodularity.

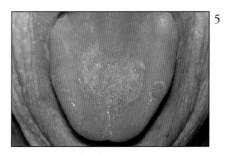

The average eruption times of each half of the upper and lower jaws are:

Deciduous:	I	C	M			Months
	7 8	18	12 24			
	6 9	18	12 24			

Permanent:	I	C	P	M		Years
	7 8	12	9 10	6 12 18+		
	7 8	12	9 10	6 12 18+		

NB: The first deciduous tooth is a lower central incisor; the first permanent tooth is a 1st molar. The lower permanent teeth appear slightly earlier than the upper. The wisdom teeth (3rd molars) appear between the 17th and 25th years and are usually the first to be shed.

The Abdomen

The anterior abdominal wall extends from the lower costal margin down to the iliac crests, inguinal ligaments and symphysis pubis. However, the cavity passes up under the rib cage to the level of the fourth intercostal space and downwards into the pelvis.

For descriptive and recording purposes the anterior abdominal wall is divided by two horizontal and two vertical lines into nine regions. The horizontal lines are the subcostal and transtubercular and the vertical lines pass through the midinguinal points, crossing the costal margins at the ninth costal cartilages. From above downwards the regions are, centrally, the epigastric, umbilical and suprapubic, and, on each side, the hypochondral, lumbar and iliac. Each lumbar region extends laterally and posteriorly into the loin.

Another useful landmark is the horizontal transpyloric plain midway between the suprasternal notch and the symphysis pubis. It crosses the body of the second lumbar vertebra, and passes through the pylorus, just above the hilum of the right kidney and just below the hilum of the left kidney. In clinical practice it is also common to refer to the quadrants of the abdomen (upper, lower, right, left) when describing the location of abnormal signs.

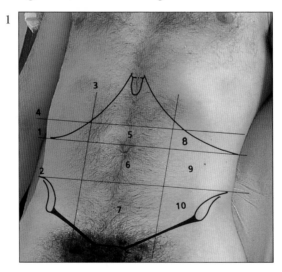

1	Regions of the abdomen	4	Transpyloric plane	8	Hypochondral
1	Subcostal line	5	Epigastrium		region
2	Transtubercular line	6	Umbilical region	9	Lumbar region
3	Midclavicular line	7	Suprapubic region	10	Iliac region

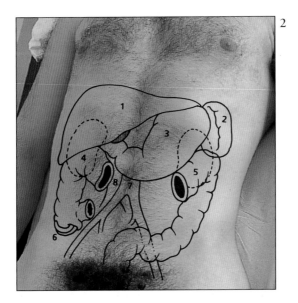

2 Abdominal viscera

1	Liver	**5**	Splenic flexure of colon
2	Spleen	**6**	Appendix
3	Stomach	**7**	Aortic bifurcation
4	Hepatic flexure of colon	**8**	Inferior vena cava

Abdominal pain is a common symptom and, in view of the large number of possible causes, it can present difficulty of diagnosis. A detailed description of the pain is essential. The site is often helpful. Epigastric pain may be related to diseases of the stomach and duodenum and is often related to meals; weight loss is a feature of gastric as well as other intra-abdominal neoplasms. Biliary pain is commonly in the right hypochondrium and radiates through to the interscapula region. Subphrenic inflammatory irritation, such as an abscess, can present with referred pain to the tip of the shoulder.

Small gut pain is characteristically around the umbilicus and may be colicky in nature, as in intestinal obstruction, and associated with disten-

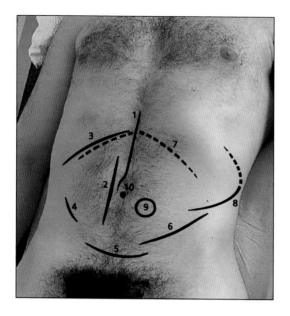

3 Abdominal incisions

1 Upper midline

2 Right paramedian

3 Kocher's incision

4 Appendicular grid iron incision

5 Suprapubic incision

6 Left iliac muscle cutting incision

7 Roof-top incision

8 Nephrectomy incision

9 Incision for terminal colostomy

10 Entry point for laparoscopic telescope

sion, vomiting and constipation. Appendicular pain often starts centrally before moving to the right iliac fossa. Severe central abdominal pain radiating through to the back may be due to acute pancreatitis, or ruptured and dissecting abdominal aortic aneurysms. In the latter check for the loss of one or both femoral pulses.

Pain and tenderness in the left iliac fossa may be due to diverticulitis or other large bowel pathology. Alteration in bowel habit in middle age and later life must be considered due to cancer until proved otherwise. Gynaecological problems, such as dysmenorrhoea, salpingitis, ruptured ovarian cyst and ectopic pregnancies, usually present with lower abdominal, often suprapubic, pain.

Renal pain is typically in the lumbar region but may radiate around to the inguinal region and scrotum, particularly incipient or obstructed hernias. Abdominal pain is further complicated by radiating pain from the chest or a nerve root.

Vomiting occurs in many abdominal conditions. Examine its contents to detect the smelly and undigested food of pyloric obstruction, or the faeculent brown fluid of intestinal obstruction. When associated with diarrhoea the vomiting may be due to gastroenteritis.

Examination of the abdomen, as in the thorax, can be considered under inspection, palpation, percussion and auscultation: inspection and palpation usually providing the most information. In this text, percussion is considered *before* palpation, since it provides useful preliminary information on tenderness and the position of organs, thus modifying the depth of palpation and showing where to palpate for the liver and spleen.

The environment must be warm and the patient relaxed, having emptied his/her bladder. He/she should lie supine with one pillow supporting the head, unless this produces dyspnoea or discomfort. Hands are placed by the sides, and the legs are extended and uncrossed. The abdomen should be fully exposed. In the male this is up to the nipples, the breasts being covered in the female. The examination must include the genitalia, but these areas are kept covered under a sheet until this part of the examination, in order not to embarrass the patient.

Inspection of the Abdomen

Note the size, shape and symmetry of the abdominal wall. These factors may be influenced by fat, a large bladder or uterus (such as in pregnancy or fibroids), distended gut, abnormal masses and ascites (free fluid). The wall may be sunken (scaphoid) in very thin patients, this being particularly so with starvation and the weight loss of malignancy. The position of the umbilicus provides information on symmetry and it may be flattened or everted and contain various amounts of debris related to the age and hygiene of the patient. It may also be the site of a hernia and congenital discharging sinuses (patent urachus). It is occasionally the site of inflammation or a metastatic nodule (Sister Joseph's nodule).

The laxity of abdominal skin is related to age and weight gain or loss. Stretch marks of pregnancy are usually laterally placed and are vertical pale scars. They may be slightly bluish, whereas those of Cushing's syndrome have a distinct purplish hue. Excessive hair in the female or absence in the male may be an indication of hormonal abnormalities, requiring examination of other secondary sexual characteristics.

The veins on the abdominal wall have no valves and may enlarge to provide collateral channels in inferior or superior vena caval obstruction and portal hypertension. They radiate from the umbilicus and, when prominent, produce the pattern termed a Caput Medusa. The application of a hot water bottle to the skin produces a characteristic mottled, faint pigmentation (erythema ab igne). These markings on the abdomen usually indicate a painful site which the patient has tried to soothe with the application of heat.

Note recent wounds, dressings, fistulae, sinuses and stomas, and the position of old scars. Ask the patient to explain each one. The abdominal wall should move freely and symmetrically in quiet (diaphragmatic) respiration. This will not be so with diaphragmatic or abdominal wall paralysis. Pain will also interfere with these movements. The restriction may be limited to one quadrant but is more widespread in generalised peritonitis, the maximum being found in perforated peptic ulcer and acute pancreatitis (p 114).

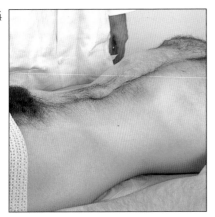
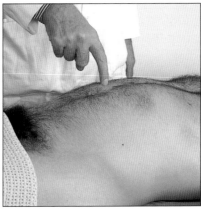

4 and 5 Ask the patient to draw his abdomen right in, and then blow it out as far as it will go. These manoeuvres will demonstrate limitation of movement due to tenderness, providing a good deal of information without any manual contact.

Coughing will accentuate these differences and will also produce pain over tender areas. On coughing, observe the abdominal wall for the presence of herniae, particularly the superficial inguinal rings, for inguinal herniae, old scars for incisional herniae, and the midline for umbilical and paraumbilical herniae, and divarication of the rectus muscles. Incisional and midline herniae are often accentuated by asking the patient to raise their head and shoulder off the bed.

Movements deep to the abdominal wall may be produced by gut peristalsis or pulsation. Pulsation is transmitted from the heart or the aorta, in a thin person, and with abnormalities such as abdominal aortic aneurysms, a mass in front of the aorta or the pulsatile liver of tricuspid incompetence. Normal gut peristalsis is occasionally seen in a very thin individual or in an incisional hernia, where the gut is covered only by skin and fascia. However visible peristalsis usually represents pathological obstruction, such as pyloric stenosis, and upper or lower intestinal obstruction, where coils of small gut produce a ladder-like writhing pattern.

The abdominal wall may bulge over normal or abnormal organs and masses, such as a pregnant uterus, an enlarged liver, spleen, bladder, ovary or gall bladder, segments of gut and mesenteric cysts. Movements and bulges can be more easily seen if the observer rests on one knee and brings his/her eyes down to the level of the anterior abdominal wall.

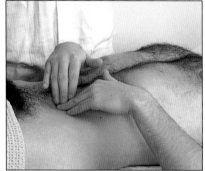

6 Finally, before proceeding to percussion and palpation, ask the patient to point out and personally palpate tender spots. This will indicate the extent to which they are willing to have their abdomen indented. This is a useful technique in children.

Percussion (see p 98)

Percussion provides a gentle means of localising abdominal tenderness, and of differentiating between solid and gaseous filled structures, thus of defining the borders of solid organs.

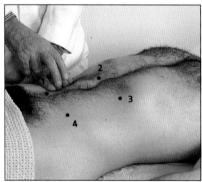
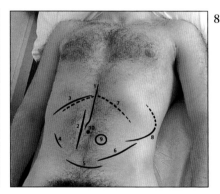

7 and 8 Commence with percussion of the four quadrants (1-4), localisation of the lower and upper borders of the liver (5, 6, 7) and spleen (8), the bladder and uterus (9) and any dullness in the flanks (10, 11). If the latter is detected it is further assessed for shifting dullness (p 117).

To look for tenderness, percuss all four quadrants leaving any known tender areas till last. The vibration of gentle percussion is sufficient to produce pain from a damaged peritoneum (percussion rebound). This form of localisation is much less painful for the patient than defining tenderness by superficial or deep palpation or by rebound tenderness (p 119). The technique is particularly useful in children. Always watch the patient's face while undertaking percussion or the palpation techniques described below.

When defining borders of organs and masses, percuss from resonant (gas filled) to dull (solid organ). The liver edge is located by percussing sequentially from the right iliac fossa to the costal margin in the right mid-clavicular line. The dullness is usually located at the costal margin but a very large liver may extend down to the right iliac fossa. Enlargement is expressed in the number of fingers or hand breadths below the costal margin. The upper edge of the liver usually reaches the 4th right intercostal space—percuss downwards in the mid-clavicular line from the second or third interspace. Hyper-resonant lung, such as in emphysema and pneumothorax, and a pneumoperitoneum, can make it difficult to locate the dullness of the upper margin.

The normal spleen is sited posterior to the left mid-axillary line and is not easily detected by percussion. It enlarges across the abdomen towards the right iliac fossa. Percussion for splenic dullness therefore starts in the right iliac fossa, passes across the umbilicus to the left costal margin at the anterior axillary line, and then along the 10th rib posteriorly. Percussion from the umbilicus down to the symphysis is usually resonant but dullness may be encountered from the upper border of an enlarging bladder, uterus or ovary, coming out of the pelvis. Abdominal masses are generally dull to percussion and alter normal patterns of resonance.

9
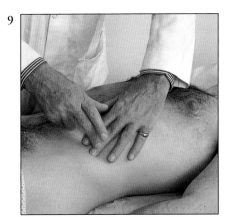
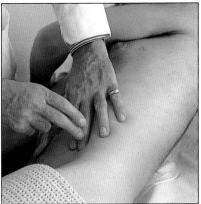
10

9 and 10 Ascites produces dullness in the flanks when lying in the supine position. Percuss from resonant to dull; moving the left hand so that the fingers remain parallel to the dull edge being sought. Note the fluid level and then rotate the patient 45 degrees to each side in turn. The abdominal wall fluid level changes since the fluid surface remains horizontal, a phenomenon known as 'shifting dullness'.

Palpation

The abdomen must not be palpated before thorough inspection or before painful sites have been identified from the history, by the patient pointing them out and by percussion. Throughout all subsequent palpation *watch the patient's face* for indications of tenderness and how the examination should proceed. Start with gentle light superficial palpation, proceed to deeper palpation of all regions and then examine specific organs, using bimanual techniques as appropriate.

Superficial Palpation

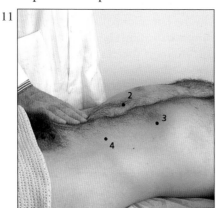

11 The examiner stands on the right side of the patient and uses the flat of the right hand, with fingers together, firm but capable of moulding to the contours of the abdominal wall. Feel each quadrant in turn. If there is a painful area, leave this till last. Some normal subjects find it difficult to relax the abdominal wall, particularly if the environment or the examiner's hands are cold, or if there is lack of privacy or any other embarrassment. Reassure the patient. Ask him to breathe deeply with his mouth open and, if necessary, to bend his knees to more than a right angle, with the feet placed flat on the couch. One is specifically looking for tenderness, guarding, rigidity and obvious masses.

On palpation, tenderness will produce local voluntary tensing (guarding) of the abdominal wall. There may also be involuntary reflex contraction (rigidity), unrelated to the external pressure or to tenderness, this indicates peritoneal inflammation (peritonism). The most extreme form is seen in the board-like rigidity often associated with a perforated peptic ulcer. In the latter it is not possible to depress any part of the abdominal wall and thumping on this board-like abdomen on any quadrant does not necessarily produce any focal tenderness. Guarding and rigidity, however, may be localised, as over an acutely inflamed appendix in the right iliac fossa or diverticulitis in the left iliac fossa.

Deep Palpation

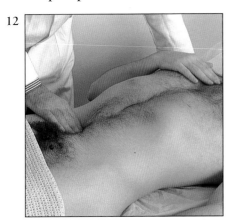

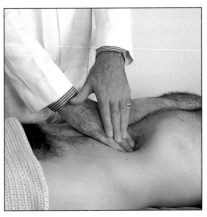

12 and 13 Each region of the abdomen must be systematically examined to identify normal and abnormal viscera and masses. A rigid, flat yet malleable right hand is again used, but placed more steeply than in gentle superficial palpation. The fingers identify the shape and size of each structure by compressing them through the lax anterior abdominal wall onto the firm posterior abdominal wall, made up of vertebral bodies and muscles. When examining a mass or a specific organ, note the size, shape, consistency and any associated tenderness.

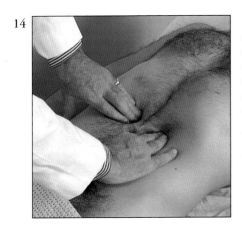

14 Both hands may be used, to measure approximate sizes of normal and abnormal viscera, to hold mobile structures and to assess expansile pulsation, by pressing on either side of the structure. As with all other aspects of abdominal palpation, watch the patient's face throughout the examination to recognise and minimize discomfort, and ensure the subject is relaxed and breathing through an open mouth.

Emphasis has already been given to the use of percussion rebound to localise tenderness. The classical method for detecting rebound tenderness is to press firmly and deeply with the hand, possibly the left hand pressing down on the back of the right, and suddenly releasing the pressure. The swing of the abdominal wall produces tension on local structures and elicits pain from any sensitive peritoneum. The method is useful in detecting mild and unsuspected tenderness. However, it must never be used when obvious tenderness exists, as it can produce severe discomfort.

The order of palpation is directed by previous information, based on the site of pain and tenderness, and abnormalities picked up on observation, percussion and gentle superficial palpation; particularly the presence of masses and herniae. It is common, after superficial palpation, to start by examining for the liver and spleen in the right and left hypochondria, then the kidneys in each flank, as described in the specific organs below. One danger is to concentrate on the four quadrants and miss midline structures such as an abdominal aortic aneurysm.

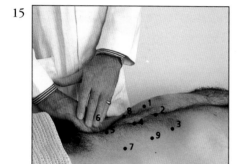

15   A possible order for routine examination (1 to 9) is from the right to the left hypochondrium, through the epigastrium, assessing the liver, the pancreas and coeliac region, the spleen and renal masses. Pass downwards to the umbilicus, to assess not only the umbilicus but the presence of aortic aneurysms and periaortic masses, and lesions of the transverse colon and stomach. Pass downwards into the suprapubic region, considering bladder, ovarian, uterine and small bowel masses, and then into each iliac fossa, with the caecum and appendix to the right and the sigmoid colon on the left. The lumbar regions are left until last (p 126). They are examined bimanually, the left hand being slid behind the region and the hands being pressed together to assess structures between, such as kidneys and the ascending and descending colon.

The site gives a strong indication of the underlying anatomy. Define the borders of the structure and whether its surface is smooth, whether it is possible to feel above, below and all around it, and whether it can be moved or moves with respiration. It may be possible to move separate masses, such as omental metastases, or decide whether a mass is within the omentum, such as a large omental cyst, or a retroperitoneal structure fixed to the posterior abdominal wall, such as a pancreatic cyst.

Abdominal masses may become more or less prominent when tensing the abdominal wall. Prominence is accentuated when a mass is superficial to the abdominal muscles, either as part of the wall or a protrusion through it, such as a hernia. The abdominal wall is tensed by coughing or asking the subject to raise his head and shoulders off the bed, without using an elbow.

When a lot of ascites is present, structures float and it is possible to bounce large structures, such as a liver or spleen, feeling them hit the posterior abdominal wall or the anterior abdominal wall on rebound: this manoeuvre is known as balloting.

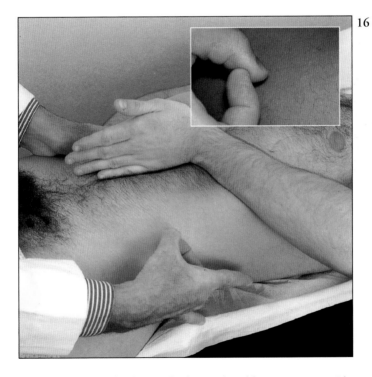

16 Vibrations of fluid may also be produced by tapping one side of the abdomen and feeling on the other. The patient or an observer places the side of a hand along the midline to prevent vibration of the anterior abdominal wall and consequent misinterpretation.

Specific Organs

Disease of a specific organ may be suspected from the history, directing attention to this viscus on examination. Suspicion may also have been raised during inspection and percussion. In a thin subject, it is not uncommon to palpate a number of normal viscera, including a smooth liver edge, the lower pole of each kidney, the caecum, the ascending, transverse and sigmoid colon, and the abdominal aorta. Other structures which may be misinterpreted as abnormal are: a long xiphisternum, which may extend to near the umbilicus, prominent rectus abdominus muscles, their intersections and divarication, and calcification in an old scar.

Liver

17

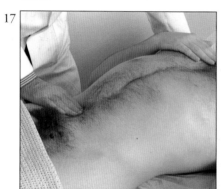

18

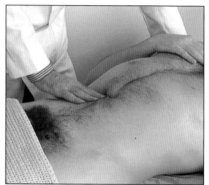

19

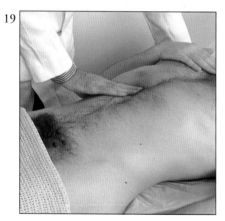

17 to 19 The liver moves downwards on inspiration and its anterior edge becomes palpable if it extends beyond the costal margin: this occasionally occurs in the normal individual. A large liver extends down towards the right iliac fossa, and the edge is often firm and easily palpable. Use the flat of the outstretched right hand, with the thumb tucked under the palm, placed at right angles to the costal margin. Press the radial border of the index finger into the abdomen during expiration and retain in this position during inspiration, when the descending edge of an enlarged liver is felt against the index finger.

Preliminary percussion will probably have indicated the lower edge of liver dullness. If in doubt start to palpate in the right iliac fossa and move upwards one or two fingers breadth at a time, until a liver edge is defined or the costal margin is reached.

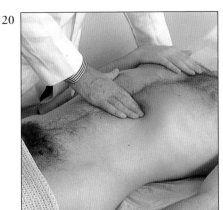

20

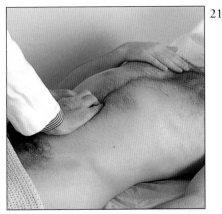

21

20 to 22 The manoeuvre is repeated to the left of the midline to detect an enlarged left lobe of the liver. An alternative technique is to use the fingertips of the two hands, placed alongside each other, parallel with the costal margin pressing inwards and upwards during inspiration, along the same pathway, or using the pulps of the fingers superiorly to detect the descending liver edge.

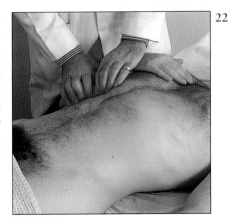

22

The liver edge is measured in finger or hand breadths below the costal margin. Note also the shape, consistency, nodularity and tenderness. A soft, one-finger breadth liver edge can be normal as may be a palpable Riedel's lobe. An enlarged left lobe may be palpable across the midline. Rectus abdominus intersections can be confused for an edge and well developed abdominal musculature can make a soft liver edge difficult to palpate.

An enlarged gall bladder extends downwards, usually as a smooth enlargement from the liver edge in the mid-clavicular line. Rolling the patient to 45 degrees on the left side increases its visibility as well as facilitating palpation. A mucocoele of the gall bladder is often palpable, but enlargement usually indicates malignant obstruction. An enlarged gall bladder may also be palpable bimanually and may be confused with a palpable right kidney, the latter being further posterior.

Tenderness over the gall bladder is present in acute cholecystitis and, with the hand depressed over the site of the gall bladder, the subject is asked to breathe in deeply. Tenderness, producing sudden stopping of inspiration, elicited in this fashion is called a positive Murphy's sign.

Spleen

The spleen enlarges from beneath the left costal margin, across the umbilicus, to the right iliac fossa. Like the liver, it descends with inspiration and the same hand movements are used to define and dip under the notched anterior margin.

23
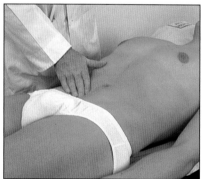

24
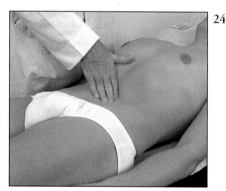

25
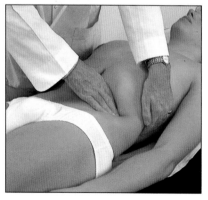

23 to 25 Palpation starts below and to the right of the umbilicus, passes upwards across the midline, and ends subcostally in the midaxillary line.

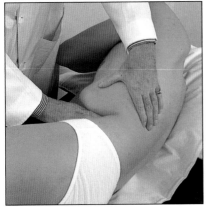 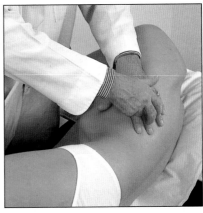

26 and 27 Palpation is facilitated by turning the patient 45 degrees to the right side and the spleen is first 'tipped' in the mid-axillary line. Normal splenic dullness should never extend beyond this point.

Epigastrium and Umbilical Regions

Stomach and pancreatic masses and aortic aneurysms are palpable in the epigastrium and behind the umbilicus. In the latter, place the finger-tips of each hand on either side of the aneurysm to demonstrate expansile pulsation and also to gain some indication of the transverse diameter (p 119). Very few aneurysms are suprarenal in origin, even when the palpating fingers cannot dip over the upper border. Aneurysms occasionally involve the common iliac arteries, in which case the aortic bifurcation may be palpable. Small aneurysms may be difficult to palpate in an obese abdomen and a normal aorta can be palpated against the vertebral bodies in a thin individual: press deeply but gently as this manoeuvre can produce discomfort.

Para-aortic nodes and fixed retroperitoneal or pancreatic masses can mimic aneurysms and may transmit aortic pulsation. A gastric neoplasm presenting as a mass in the epigastrium or umbilical region may be partly mobile in all directions. In the neonate, the pyloric tumour of pyloric stenosis may be palpable, after a meal, on the right side of the epigastrium.

Suprapubic Region

The suprapubic region is usually resonant and empty to palpation. The commonest mass coming out of the pelvis, which one cannot get below and is dull to percussion, is the pregnant uterus. A large bladder and ovarian masses can have similar signs, in the former, the patient usually has accompanying urinary difficulties.

The Colon

This may be palpated in most of its course when loaded with solid or semi-solid faecal material or if it is distended, as in intestinal obstruction. It is often smooth, ill defined and sausage shaped, with some side to side mobility. The contents may be indented. The caecum, in the right iliac fossa, is more rounded.

The transverse colon dips across the epigastrium and umbilical regions. The sigmoid colon passes across the left iliac fossa, descending into the pelvis. It is commonly felt in thin individuals and can be identified by the indentible faecal content. The ascending and descending portions of the colon can be felt in the right and left lumbar regions by direct palpation or bimanually (see below).

Lumbar Regions

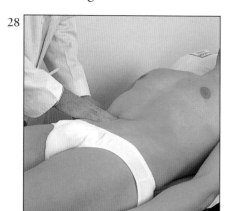

28

28 The contents of the lumbar regions are best felt bimanually. The left hand is placed behind the loin, in line with the right, and the two hands pressed together.

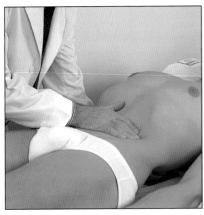

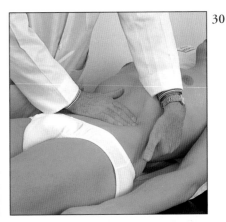

30

29 to 31 To examine the left lumbar region, the left hand is either passed across behind the subject's back or the examiner leans over the subject to slide the hand behind the loin. Rolling the patient onto the opposite side may also facilitate palpation.

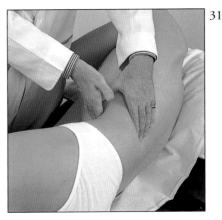

31

Renal tenderness is usually maximum posteriorly. The kidneys descend on inspiration and may be felt between the two hands. The lower poles may be palpable in normal subjects, particularly that of the lower placed right kidney. A large low-lying or mobile kidney may be caught between the two hands, and felt to recoil when let go.

A renal mass may be resonant to percussion, due to overlying colonic gas. A colonic mass is more anteriorly placed and may be dull to percussion.

Auscultation

Normal gut sounds may be audible even without a stethoscope, particularly after meals and with hunger. At other times sounds may be remarkably few, occurring up to every 10 seconds. These borborygmi (gurgles) can be best heard by placing the stethoscope to the right of the umbilicus. The sounds are markedly accentuated in intestinal obstruction, particularly during the contractions of a colic. They are also increased by irritation from blood in the bowel or in any form of diarrhoea.

Excess fluid in the gut, as for example in pyloric stenosis, may splash around when the abdomen in gently shaken by holding either side of the pelvis. This 'succussion splash' may also be present two to three hours after a meal. It may be audible without a stethoscope. If not, ask the patient to hold the instrument in position.

Paralysed gut, such as post-operatively or in generalised peritonitis, is silent. But listen intently for a few minutes. In the late stages of intestinal obstruction, the gut may be markedly dilated and atonic, with few gut sounds but with marked hyper-resonance (a condition known as tympanitic) with tinkling sounds of fluid dripping from one distended loop to another. In complete paralysis, breath and heart sounds may be clearly audible over the abdomen.

A peritoneal rub is produced by friction between roughened peritoneal surfaces, such as in inflammation and neoplasia. They disappear if the surfaces adhere or the condition improves. Rubs over liver abscesses and splenic infarcts may be misinterpreted as arising from a pleural rub of pulmonary disease.

32

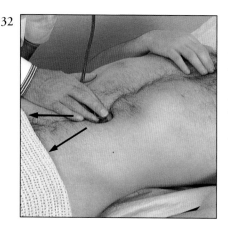

32 Bruits may be heard in the epigastrium down to the umbilicus and onwards to each mid-inguinal point in aorto-iliac arterial stenotic disease. Increased porta-systemic flow in portal hypertension may produce venous sounds, these being increased on inspiration and during a Valsalva manoeuvre.

33 Renal artery bruits may be more audible posteriorly. The patient is turned onto his right side. While in this position splenic dullness can be percussed and the spleen and left kidney palpated. Sacral oedema may also be noted (p 82).

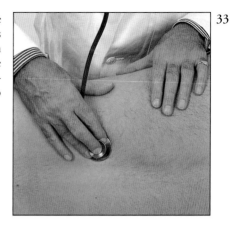

33

Abdominal veins may be present over a normal abdominal wall. They are particularly prominent, radiating from the umbilicus in portal venous obstruction.

34

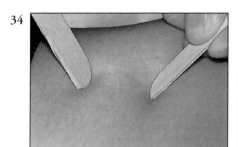

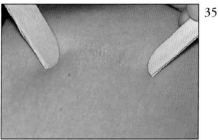

35

34 and 35 The direction of blood flow in the vein can be obtained by using a finger or some other implement to compress one end. Express the blood out of a segment and then release the first compression point to see if the flow is towards the second compression point. The procedure is repeated in the opposite direction and over different veins across the abdomen.

The Inguinal Region and Perineum

Groins and Genitalia

The abdominal examination is completed by exposure and full examination of the inguinal regions—the scrotum and penis in the male and the perineum in the female. Although the anterior superior iliac spines are palpable, the pubic tubercles and symphysis pubis may be difficult to palpate in obese subjects.

The inguinal ligament extends from the anterior superior iliac spine to the pubic tubercle. Direct and indirect inguinal herniae extrude through the superficial inguinal ring, above and medial to the pubic tubercle. Inguinal herniae often reduce spontaneously in the supine position, but can usually be seen to reappear on asking the patient to cough.

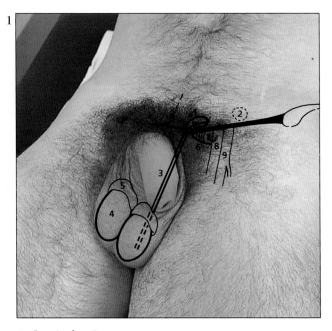

1 Inguinal region

1 Superficial inguinal ring	**6** Lacunar ligament
2 Deep inguinal ring	**7** Neck of femoral canal
3 Vas deferens	**8** Femoral vein
4 Testis	**9** Femoral artery
5 Superior pole of epididymis	

2 Place the middle and ring fingers over the superficial inguinal ring and ask the patient to cough again. The gut can be felt to extrude through the ring. This has to be differentiated from tensing of the abdominal wall and the slight bulging of the supra-inguinal region just lateral to the tubercle, often present in normal individuals and termed a Malgaigne's bulge.

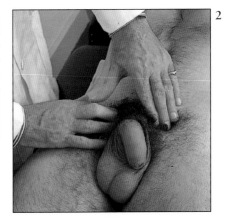

2

3 If a hernia is not obvious the patient is asked to stand up and cough again. If there is still doubt ask the subject to don some clothes, and walk and climb some stairs, but on return to remain standing until examined in this position again.

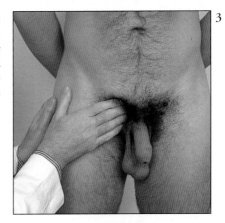

3

4 In the male it is possible to invaginate the upper part of the scrotum superiorly subcutaneously into the superficial inguinal ring, even in an obese patient, and the cough impulse of a hernial sac to be felt. This manoeuvre, however, must be undertaken very gently, as it may cause discomfort, and the invagination of the scrotum must start low enough to follow the line of the spermatic cord, deep to subcutaneous fat.

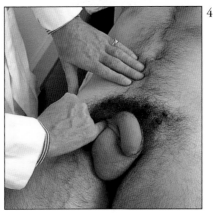

4

Once a hernia has been found it is important to be sure that it is reducible and, once reduced, to differentiate between direct and indirect inguinal hernia by seeing if the cough impulse can be controlled by pressure over the deep inguinal ring. Whether this is tested in the lying or standing position depends on the ease of reducing and reproducing the hernia by coughing. The deep inguinal ring is situated just above the midpoint of the inguinal ligament. The finger is placed over this site after hernia reduction, and asking the subject to cough, either in the standing or lying position, depending on how the hernia is most easily reproduced. Both inguinal regions must be examined, even if a patient is complaining of just a unilateral lump, since the condition is often bilateral.

A number of structures produce masses below the inguinal ligament. Common findings are inguinal lymph nodes (p 53) and femoral herniae. The latter appear below and lateral to the pubic tubercle; they are usually more difficult to reduce than their inguinal counterparts. A tender, irreducible hernia is difficult to differentiate from a tender lymph node in this region. Other lumps include a saphenous varix, a femoral aneurysm and abscesses.

Scrotum

The scrotum contains, on each side, the testes, epididymis and the contents of the spermatic cord. An indirect inguinal hernia may follow the spermatic cord into the scrotum.

5

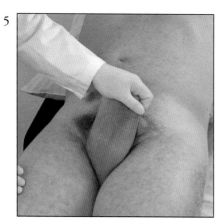

5 Examination is usually in the lying position. In the male, ask the patient to spread his legs to allow the scrotum to be raised onto the front of the thighs. This can be done by pulling on the inferior scrotal skin, but do not hold the testes during this movement, as it is painful. Examine the skin of the posterior as well as the anterior surface of the scrotum. Note the distribution of hair around the pubis and scrotum and any skin abnormality.

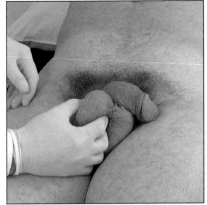
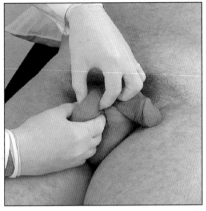

6 and 7 Examine the contents of the scrotum one side at a time. The testis is sensitive to pressure and during gentle palpation observe the subject's face. Check the oval, vertical orientation of the normal 3cm adult testis with superior, posterior and inferior epididymis and the vas deferens passing cranially behind the testis from the inferior pole.

8 The spermatic cord is palpated at the neck of the scrotum where the contents can be rolled between finger and thumb, the prominent vas deferens being palpable. It is at this site that the vas deferens is manipulated to a subcutaneous position for the operation of vasectomy.

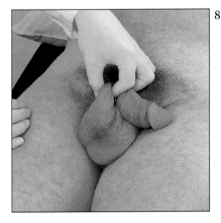

8

If a scrotal mass is present, first decide whether it is possible to get above it. If not, the inguinoscrotal extension is probably an indirect inguinal hernia. If the mass is confined to the scrotum, check whether the testis can be palpated as a discrete entity or whether it is surrounded by the mass, this being the case in a hydrocele. The latter may be tensely filled with fluid and the testes difficult to palpate. Cysts of the epididymus are usually sited above the testis and can be palpated separate from it, although occasionally they may occur within a hydrocele sac.

Swellings of the testis may be neoplastic, often presenting as focal swellings with reduced sensitivity to gentle pressure. Other swellings include infection; acute infections often cause enlargement of the testis and epididymis. Congenital anomalies include small or absent testes or horizontally lying testes. The latter are more prone to torsion, particularly if the epididymis is not firmly applied to the side as well as the two ends of the testes.

9

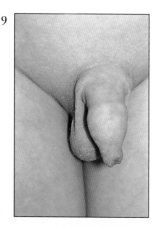

9 The prepubertal testis and epididymus are the same shape as the adult. Note the absence of secondary sexual hair development.

10

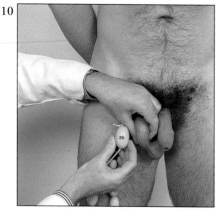

10 Testicular size is assessed by comparison with a standard size set of oval beads.

Separation of cystic and solid structures is aided by transillumination. A varicocele is a collection of varicosities (of the pampiniform plexus) which has been aptly described as a 'bag of worms'.

134

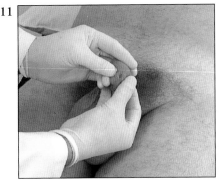

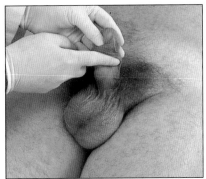

11 When examining the penis note whether the subject has been circumcised (compare the figure with the uncircumcised penis, p 131). If not, retract the foreskin to ensure there is no underlying lesion and check the normality of the urethral orifice. Always replace the retracted foreskin to avoid risk of a paraphimosis.

12 When examining a patient for venereal disease, the penile urethra is massaged from proximal to distal to express and sample any urethral discharge.

Rectal and Vaginal Examination

The abdominal examination is completed by examination of the perineum, including rectal, and sometimes vaginal, examination, these usually being undertaken with the subject in the left lateral position.

13 Rectal examination provides valuable information on pelvic organs. Explain the importance of the procedure to the patient, who should turn onto the left side, so the pelvis is a true vertical, bringing the buttocks to the edge of the couch and drawing the knees up to the chest: ensure adequate lighting to observe the perineum. Put on a pair of disposable gloves and first lift up the right buttock to expose the anus, the back of the scrotum or the vaginal margins. Note any abnormality of the skin, protrusions from the anal canal or other lesions. Ask the patient to strain down and note any extrusion of skin or mucosa through the anus.

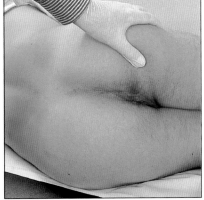

13

14

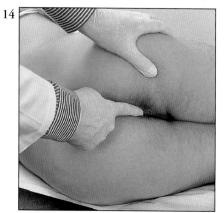

14 Dip the gloved right index finger into a lubricant and lubricate the anal margin. Tell the subject that you are intending to insert the finger. Rest the pulp of the finger on the anal margin and gently curl the tip into the anus. Proceed slowly and note any tenderness or spasm as the finger passes through the anal sphincter. Extreme tenderness and spasm may indicate a fissure and may prevent further examination unless carried out very slowly and very gently. Usually the finger passes easily through the sphincter into the anal canal and the lower rectum. Note any surrounding lumps or nodularity within the anal canal.

15

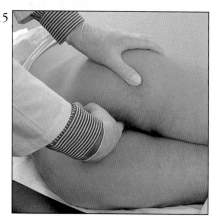

15 Systematically examine the contents of the pelvis. First feel the hollow of the sacrum and the coccyx, which may be examined between the finger inside and the thumb outside.

16

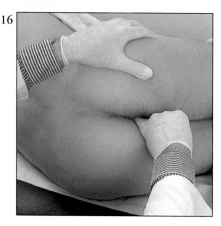

16 Turn the hand anticlockwise round the left side of the pelvis to examine anteriorly. In a normal prostate, the groove between the two lateral lobes is palpable. The seminal vesicles lie above this but are not usually palpable. The tip of the finger however is touching the peritoneum of the pouch of Douglas, through the wall of the rectum, and will detect abnormalities within the pouch, including the tenderness of pelvic peritonitis.

The finger is further rotated to examine the right side of the pelvis and the patient requested to strain down as the finger negotiates the lower rectum to note any abnormality of the wall.

17 Further information may be obtained by bimanual examination, the left hand palpating the lower abdomen. A common anal abnormality is protrusion of the skin and mucosa of the anal canal through the external sphincter, a condition known as haemorrhoids or piles.

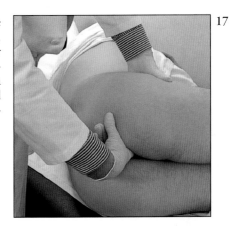

17

In the female, anteriorly is the vagina. The rounded firm cervix with a central canal can be felt through the rectal wall. Lean over the patient and rest the left hand over the suprapubic region to examine the pelvis bimanually, when it may be possible to assess the shape and size of the uterus, and any associated abnormalities.

Note any tenderness in the fornices, suggesting pelvic inflammatory disease. The ovaries lie on the lateral wall and are not usually palpable but may become so in the presence of an ovarian cyst.

Note the presence of faecal material in the rectum and, on removal of the finger, note the consistency of this material and the existence of any blood or mucus on the glove before disposing of it. Clean the anus with toilet paper then ask the patient to return to the supine position.

Vaginal examination produces additional information on the cervix, uterus, fornices and ovaries after preliminary examination of the vulva and introitus. This does not form part of routine abdominal examination, but is included as part of a gynaecological examination and when it is thought additional information on pelvic abnormalities can be obtained. It may be carried out in the left lateral position or in the supine position with the knees bent to a right angle and the hips abducted. This position is of particular value when carrying out bimanual examination of the female genital tract.

Abnormal findings may also lead to further examination by proctoscopy and sigmoidoscopy and the use of a vaginal speculum.

Checklist for the Assessment of the Alimentary and Genitourinary Systems

History

Weight (current, changes); fatigue; pigmentation

Pain: site, radiation, relation to food

Flatulence; nausea; vomiting; haematemesis

Dysphagia: site, solids/fluids

Stool: frequency, quantity, consistency, mucus, blood (fresh, altered, melaena), tenesmus

Perianal pain; lumps; discharge; pruritus

Micturition: frequency; nocturia; polyuria; oliguria; haematuria; obstruction; hesitancy; poor stream; dribbling; urgency; dysuria

Urethral discharge/pain

Urine: amount, discoloration, clarity, colour, blood, debris

Menstruation: menarche, menopause, dysmenorrhoea, menorrhagia, amenorrhoea

Dyspareunia: superficial/deep; vaginal discharge; contraception

Pregnancy: last menstrual period; expected date of delivery; abdominal pain; haemorrhage; venous thrombosis

Examination

General—NB: presence and features of any vomitus
Encephalopathy; weight loss; obesity; cachexia; dehydration; hypo/hyper pigmentation

Hands: palmar flush; telangectasia; Dupuytren's contracture; skin laxity; muscle wasting; arthropathy; liver flap

Nails: pallor; clubbing; spooning; leukonychia; onycholysis

Head and neck: conjunctival pallor; jaundice; xanthelasma; halitosis (hepatic, uraemic, faecal, ketotic); tongue (dry, furred, glossitis, leukoplakia); gingivitis; dentition

Cervical lymphadenopathy (NB: scalene node)

Salivary glands: tenderness and swelling

Abdomen

Lying supine with a single pillow, fully exposed but breasts and genitalia covered until these areas are examined

Inspection

Skin: laxity; pigmentation; bruising; scratch marks; stria; hair distribution; scars; sinuses; fistulae; stomas; dilated veins; herniae; divarication of the recti

Umbilicus: position, hygiene, nodules, discharge

Distension; scaphoid abdomen; respiratory movements; visible peristalsis

Enlarged organs: liver, gall bladder, spleen, uterus; masses

Discomfort on blowing out/drawing in abdominal wall and coughing

Percussion

Four quadrants, examining for rebound tenderness, hyper-resonance and the position of organs (liver, spleen, bladder, uterus), masses, ascites, shifting dullness

Palpation

NB: watch patient's face throughout. In tender abdomens and in children start with self-examination to identify tender areas

Superficial/deep four quadrant: tenderness, guarding, rigidity

Organs: liver, gall bladder, spleen, kidneys, bladder, uterus, colon/faeces

Masses: stomach, pancreas, uterus, ovarian, large/small bowel; retroperitoneal

Aorto-iliac aneurysms

Ballottable organs/masses; fluid thrill; sacral oedema

Auscultation

Gut sounds: normal, absent, tinkling, increased

Friction rubs

Renal, aorto-iliac bruits/hums

Succussion splash

Inguinal/Femoral Hernia

If not obvious ask the patient to stand

Inspection

Site; overlying skin; cough impulse

Palpation

Reduction by patient; tenderness, cough impulse, reducibility, anatomical position of neck, controllability

Inguinal/axillary nodes

External Genitalia

Draw scrotum onto the front of the thighs

Inspection

Symmetry, skin, scars, rashes

Swellings: inguino-scrotal, scrotal (testis, epididymis)

Palpation

Testis; epididymis; spermatic cord

Relation of cyst/masses to testis/epididymis

Penis: circumcised; retractable foreskin; position and shape of meatus; balanitis; discharge

Rectal/Vaginal examinations

The Nervous System

The collection and grouping of symptoms facilitate anatomical localization of lesions within the central and peripheral nervous systems. Cerebration can be altered in psychiatric as well as organic disease and its various components, such as behaviour, emotion, thought process and intelligence, are considered under the psychiatric assessment (p 23).

Of particular note in the neurological history are disturbances of consciousness, speech, memory, and motor and sensory function. Headache is a common symptom, particularly in raised intracranial pressure, but it lacks specificity since it occurs in many other complaints.

Note the frequency, timing, duration and progress of symptoms, and what the patient was doing at the time of onset of faints, falls or fits. Epilepsy may be accompanied by tongue biting and urinary incontinence. Associated chest pain, palpitations or dyspnoea may indicate a cardiac or respiratory aetiology for these symptoms.

Speech disturbances are primarily due to abnormalities of articulation (dysarthria and anarthria) or of the organization of language (dysphasia, aphasia). The muscles of the palate, tongue, larynx and pharynx have bilateral cortical innervation.

Thus disturbances of articulation require damage to a lower motor neurone (cranial nerve), the nucleus (bulbar palsy) or bilateral upper motor neurone damage (pseudobulbar palsy). Basal ganglia disease produces slow and monotonous speech, whereas cerebellar disorders characteristically produce staccato or scanning speech.

Damage to Broca's area (precentral cortex of the dominant hemisphere) produces an expressive dysphasia, the patient knowing what to say but unable to produce words. Mild degrees present as failure to name common objects and names (nominal aphasia). These conditions are commonly accompanied by inability to write (agraphia).

Dysphasia may also be produced by lesions of the parietal region due to failure of understanding of the spoken or written word (receptive aphasia, word deafness and word blindness). If Broca's area is not affected the subject may produce a stream of disconnected words (jargon aphasia). More commonly, extensive lesions affect the expression as well as the understanding of speech (global aphasia).

Disturbances of memory may be short or long term; the former is frequently due to organic disease and may be reversible.

Motor symptoms include paralysis, spasticity, incoordination and abnormal movements. Mild paresis may present with fatigue and weakness, such as diminution of grip and toe catching when walking. Spasticity may be due to pyramidal or extrapyramidal disease. In milder forms it presents with stiffness.

Cerebellar dysfunction interferes with everyday activities such as writing and eating or may produce a mild intension tremor and loss of balance. Abnormal movements include the tremor of Parkinson's disease, tics and choreiform movements.

The distribution of the sensory disturbances of paraesthesia (pins and needles), numbness, increased sensation (hyperaesthesia) and pain, provide important information on the localization of lesions; visceral pain may be referred to somatic dermatomes.

Neurological Examination

Neurological examination may be a detailed assessment of disease of the nervous system following up a specific symptom, or a survey of the system as part of a routine general examination. A detailed neurological examination can be time consuming and exhausting for a patient and information obtained from a tired, fatigued, uncooperative or ill patient can be misleading. Initial examination should therefore be targeted on the suspected abnormality, such as a peripheral nerve injury, going back one or more times to complete the observations. Follow up of neurological findings is critical when abnormalities have been found or are suspected.

Diseases may affect single cortical areas, spinal tracts or peripheral nerves but lesions often involve more than one pathway. Localization of the disease is helped by a precise history. However, it is important to keep an open mind, as it is easy to follow a wrong lead as to the level of a lesion and be blinkered about the possibility of disease at other levels or at multiple sites.

One gains an overall impression of neurological function from the patient's gait, posture and speech, but this account initially considers examination of the cranial nerves followed by assessment of motor and sensory function. Examination of the current mental state is considered under psychiatric assessment, but a few simple tests should be applied. These include orientation in time and place (what are the day and date, where are you), short and long term memory (repeat three to five words or numbers and request again after a short interval; birthday, place of birth, anniversaries); general knowledge, (names of presidents, ministers, capitals); mathematical skills (take 7's from 100); interpretation of proverbs.

Cranial Nerves

1 The olfactory (first) nerves of each side are tested in turn by compressing the contralateral nostril and applying preparations such as cloves, peppermint and a fetid odour. Pungent preparations, such as ammonia, should be avoided as these also stimulate the fifth nerve and may be misinterpreted. More sophisticated tests require dilution of the odorant to determine threshold levels.

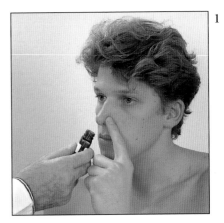

Optic (second) nerve tests encompass visual acuity, colour and visual fields, together with the visual component of pupillary reflexes.

Distant vision is assessed with Snellen Charts (p 29). Two numbers are reported. The first is the distance of the subject from the chart in metres (usually 6). The chart has 8 rows of letters which can be seen with the normal eye at respectively 60, 36, 24, 18, 12, 8, 6 and 5 metres away. The second number reported is the distance of the smallest line that can be seen. At 6 metres, this is usually the 7th line and the reported vision is 6/6 for the tested eye. If the acuity is less than 6/60, the subject is moved towards the chart (eg 3/60). If the top line cannot be read at one metre (i.e. worse than 1/60) acuity is reported as counting fingers (CF), seeing hand movements (HM) or perception of light (PL).

2 Near vision is assessed with J Charts of different size prints, each with an assigned code. Colour vision is assessed with an Ishihara Chart. This has the pattern outlined in colours in an otherwise uniform format.

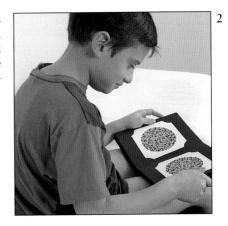

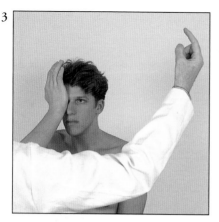

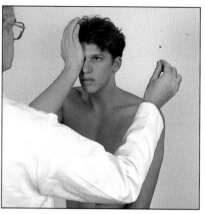

3 and 4 Clinical assessment of the visual field is by confrontation; the observer sits or stands in front of the subject and both cover one opposing eye with a palm. The subject fixates on the bridge of the examiner's nose. The examiner then brings a moving finger, or more sensitively a red headed pen, from outside his/her visual field radially inwards from each quadrant in turn.

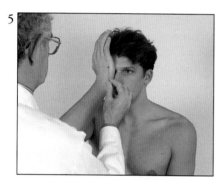

5 A central target is used to identify a scotoma (loss of central field). The subject is asked to say as soon as the finger is noted, or in the case of the pin, the red colour is identified. The examiner compares this with his/her own observation (assuming he has normal vision).

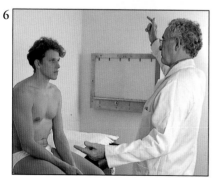

6 Visual inattention defects are assessed by the examiner moving fingers of both hands, separately or together, the subject being asked to identify which finger(s) move.

A more precise mapping of the peripheral fields and of the blind spot are obtained using perimetry. The subject's head is placed, by a chin rest, in the centre of the apparatus. This allows a light to be brought in from all directions. Alternatively, the Bjerrum screen is used, a white or red disc being moved radially inwards against a black background. Loss of parts of the visual field and loss of nasal or temporal fields, such as damage to the optic radiation or pituitary tumours pressing on the optic chiasm, can be accurately mapped.

7

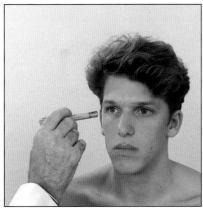

8

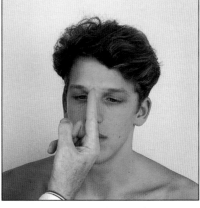

7 Direct light reflexes are tested with a pen torch, examining each eye in turn. Pupillary contraction is noted in the stimulated and the contralateral eye (consensual response).

8 The accommodation reflex is assessed by asking the patient to fixate on a distant object and then on a finger placed close to the bridge of the nose. It may be necessary to retract the eyelid to better visualize the pupil. The shape of the pupils may be altered by adhesions from local disease, and the pupillary response by neurological disorders.

9

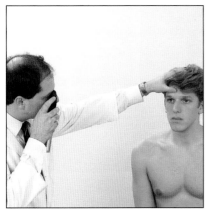

9 By observing the retina from a distance through an ophthalmoscope, one should see a red central disc (red reflex). This is disturbed by opacities within the lens, or of the aqueous or vitreous humour.

145

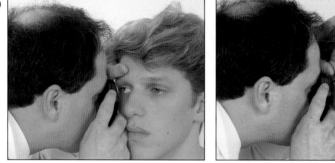

10 and 11 Observation of the retina using an ophthalmoscope begins with the subject looking straight ahead and then to each position of gaze.

Nine positions of gaze

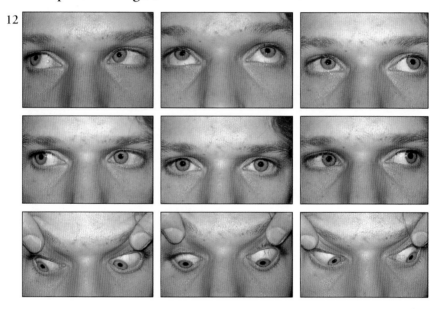

12 Positions of gaze testing cranial nerves 3, 4 and 6. The subject is intially requested to look straight ahead, note being taken of any discongugate gaze (squint).

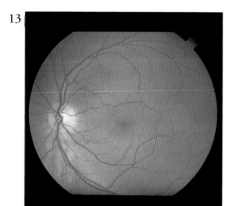

13   The normal retina seen through an ophthalmoscope. The pale optic disc is the site of entry of the optic nerve and vessels radiate from this point, branching dichotomously. The arteries are brighter red and slightly narrower than the veins. The disc is insensitive to light and is termed the 'blind spot'. The macula is the central part of the back of the retina. Lateral to the disc, it is largely devoid of vessels but has a rich capillary network. The central depression is the fovea centralis, where visual resolution is highest.

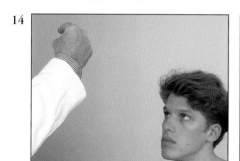 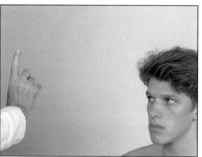

14 and 15 Normal eye movements are demonstrated by asking the subject to follow the examiner's finger, moving up and down and then from side to side, the finger following an H shape. Note any nystagmus (most commonly horizontal flicking of the eye medially from the lateral extreme gaze) to each side, whether there is double vision in any direction of gaze, any squint or any defect in eye movement.

In third (*oculomotor*) nerve palsy, the eye is displaced downwards and outwards. With ptosis (drooping of the upper lid), the only movement is further outwards and a little downwards. The defect, however, is often only partial and the diagnosis is supported by normal fourth and sixth nerve function.

In fourth (*trochlear*) nerve palsy the eye does not move outwards beyond the midline optical axis.

Although the superior oblique muscle acting independently turns the pupil downwards and outwards, its most powerful movement is in downward gaze. The oblique end of the muscle is in line with the optical axis, and produces its maximum force, when the pupil is turned inwards by other optic muscles. The sixth (*abducent*) nerve is therefore tested by asking the subject to look downwards and inwards, noting failure of downward gaze.

Detecting an abnormality of nerve function can be complicated if the underlying defect is primarily muscular, such as in thyrotoxicosis or myasthenia gravis, as these defects may affect individual muscles selectively.

A Horner's syndrome (from damage to the cervical sympathetic chain) produces ptosis, meiosis (small pupil), enophthalmos (sunken eye), failure of sweating on the ipsilateral face and stuffiness of the ipsilateral nasal cavity.

16
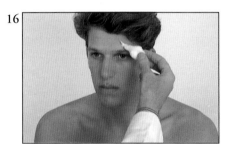

17
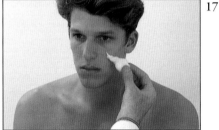

18
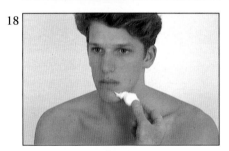

16 to 18 Touch, pain and temperature are tested (see p 155) over the temple, cheek and jaw, corresponding to the ophthalmic, maxillary and mandibular divisions of the trigeminal (fifth) cranial nerve.

19
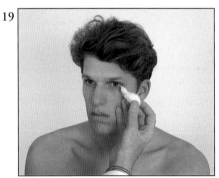

19 To test the corneal reflex, twist the corner of a piece of cotton wool into a point. Ask the subject to look towards the other side, then stroke the cotton wool gently over the exposed cornea. Be sure not to touch the eyelashes and remain out of the line of vision. Note any contact lenses; ask the subject to remove them when testing this reflex. The muscles controlling the positive blink reflex are innervated by the seventh nerve, the sensory component being the trigeminal.

20 Taste in the anterior two thirds of the tongue is carried with the seventh nerve by the chorda tympani from the mandibular division of the trigeminal nerve. Dampen three cotton wool buds in tap water and, after dipping them respectively into salt, sugar and vinegar, assess recognition of each modality on each side of the tongue. Loss of taste is termed ageusia.

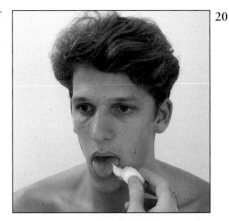

21 and 22 The motor fibres of the trigeminal nerve supply the muscles of mastication. Ask the subject to bite hard and palpate the contracting masseter and temporalis muscles over the angle of the jaw and the temple respectively.

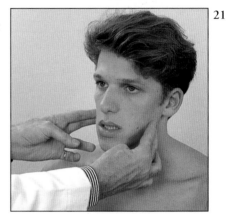

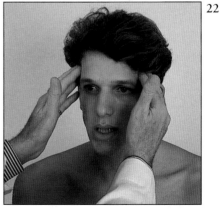

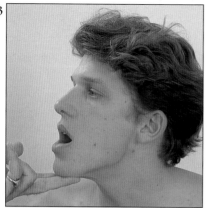

23 Protrusion of the jaw is by the pterygoid muscles and can be assessed against resistance.

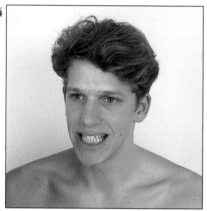

24 and 25 The *facial* (seventh) nerve innervates the muscles of facial expression. Note expression and its symmetry at rest, during talking and when smiling. In particular note the symmetry of the nasolabial folds and the angles of the mouth. Ask the subject to close his eyes, show his teeth and to whistle.

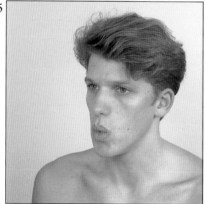

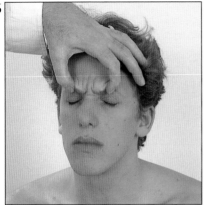

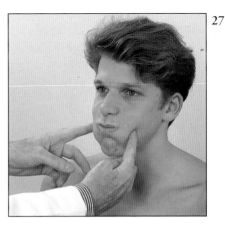

25

26 and 27 The power of the facial muscles can be assessed by trying to open the tightly screwed up eye and squashing blown out cheeks.

(The taste fibres of the facial nerve, transferred by the chorda tympani to the trigeminal nerve, are considered on page 149.)

28 Assessment of auditory function of the *vestibulocochlear* (eighth) nerve is with a whisper or a watch ticking in each ear, having checked that there is no wax interfering with air conduction.

28

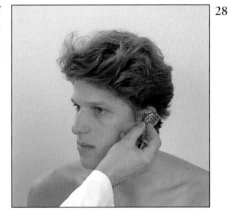

29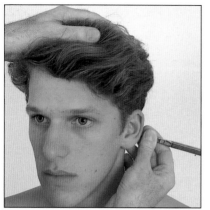

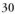30

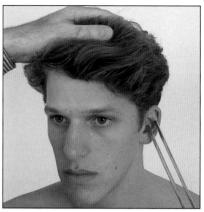

29 and 30 Air conduction should be better than bone conduction. Therefore, if the base of a vibrating tuning fork is placed over the mastoid process and the subject is asked to say as soon as the vibration stops, turning the vibrating fork near the ear should be accompanied by return of sound; this is known as Rinne's test. If the sound does not return, the implication is that bony conduction is better than air and may indicate damage to the tympanic membrane or disease of the middle ear.

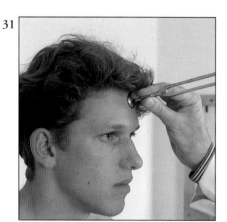

31 Comparing the two sides is by Weber's test in which the base of a vibrating tuning fork is placed over the middle of the forehead and the subject is asked whether it is heard more distinctly in one ear than the other. The fork is normally heard centrally, but may be lateralised, e.g. in the presence of middle ear disease.

A more precise assessment of hearing is with audiometry, applying different noise levels at different frequencies and recording the responses. The balance component of the nerve is assessed by running cold water into each ear in turn. A positive response produces nystagmus towards the stimulated side.

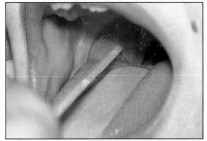

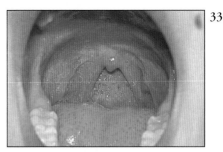

33

32 The *glossopharyngeal* (ninth) nerve innervates the stylopharyngeus muscle; this cannot be tested independently. Sensation is over the tonsil and anterior pillar of the fauces. Examination is by the gag reflex produced by gently touching the anterior pillar with a wooden spatula. Taste over the posterior third of the tongue is assessed as with the trigeminal nerve, but this area is more sensitive to bitter tastes, such as quinine.

33 The motor component of the *vagus* (tenth) nerve produces movement of the soft palate and with the *accessory* (eleventh), produces swallowing and speech. The position of the uvula can be unreliable but ask the patient to say 'ah' to assess symmetry. Observe or gently palpate the larynx while the patient is swallowing a glass of water (p 45), and note the pitch and power of speech.

Laryngeal and pharyngeal muscles are bilaterally innervated and dysarthria and dysphagia require lower motor neurone or bilateral upper motor neurone denervation (see p 141). Unilateral damage to the recurrent laryngeal nerve, which may be produced by neoplasia or surgery of the thyroid gland, interferes with coughing (producing a bovine cough without the explosive element produced by tight apposition of the vocal cords) and the subject is unable to sing a high pitched 'ee'.

34 The cervical component of the accessory nerve innervates sternomastoid and trapezius muscles, the latter being assessed by shrugging of the shoulders against resistance.

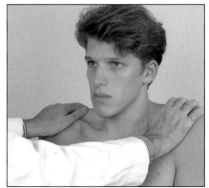

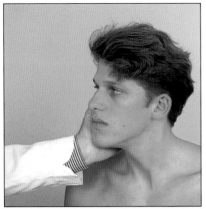

34

35 Place the palm of the hand against the right side of the subject's jaw and ask him/her to turn the head to the right against this resistance while observing and feeling the left sterno-mastoid muscle. Repeat the procedure for the right.

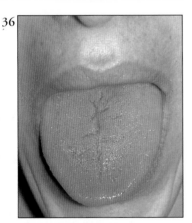

36 The *hypoglossal* (twelfth) nerve innervates the intrinsic and extrinsic muscles of the tongue. Denervation is accompanied by wasting of the ipsilateral side and weakness of movement towards this side. Movements are assessed by rapid pointing and withdrawing of the tongue and during speech.

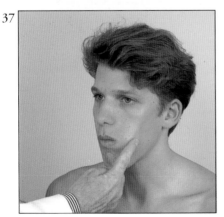

37 Power is assessed by pushing the tongue against resistance applied to the outside of the cheek.

Sensory Function

Somatic Sensation

Altered sensation varies from absence to excess (hyperaesthesia). Be sure the patient is not using the term 'numbness' to describe limb weakness. Ask the patient to outline any abnormal area of sensation. Another point of possible misinterpretation is to label sensory inattention as sensory loss. In the former patients may require a good deal of verbal encouragement to pay attention during the examination.

In examination of an asymptomatic patient, examine the limb extremities first: if these are normal, it is not usually necessary to examine more proximally in detail. During sensory examination, expose the area of interest, together with the equivalent parts of the opposite side of the body.

Observation of the skin provides information on sensory innervation before examining each sensory modality. Insensitive skin is susceptible to damage from unnoticed minor trauma. An extreme example is in leprosy, where the long term sequelae is loss of digits.

1 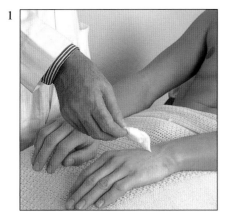 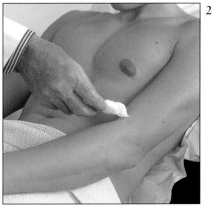 2

1 and 2 *Touch and light pressure* are transmitted in the dorsal columns to the postcentral cortex. Initially they are tested by finger contact over the affected area. More detailed mapping is with a wisp of cotton wool or an artist's paintbrush. Let the patient watch while the stimulus is applied, to ensure a positive response is appreciated, and compare it with the contralateral side.

When examining an abnormal area, ask the patient to close his eyes and say 'yes' every time contact is made. When looking for changes in sensation, ask whether each stimulus is normal or abnormal. Move from insensitive to normal areas or from normal to hyperaesthetic, varying the rate and the rhythm of the stimuli. Gently mark the boundaries of change with a biro or skin pencil. This enables the examiner to check consistency of response and also to reproduce these markings in diagrammatic form.

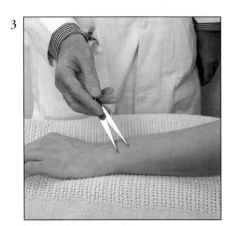

3 Two blunt points are distinguished as separate contacts at varying distances in different parts of the body: lips and tongue 2–3mm; fingertips 3–5mm; dorsum of fingers 4–6mm; palm 8–15mm; dorsum of hand 20–30mm; dorsum of feet 30–40mm; back 40–50mm.

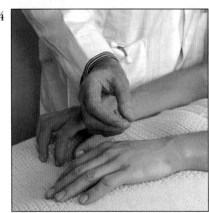

4 *Pain and temperature* are carried to the level of sensory awareness in the spinothalmic tracts. The former is tested with a sterile pin or a partially blunted 21 gauge needle, the patient being asked to respond to each contact, stating whether dull or sharp.

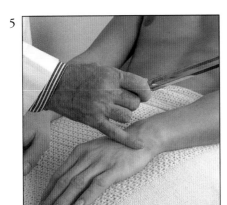

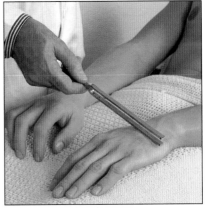

5 and 6 For gross temperature differences, compare the warmth of the outer side of the little finger with the cold of the side of a tuning fork. More precise mapping is with test tubes of cold and warm water. Temperature changes may be more consistent than those of pinprick. Mapping follows the same routine to that described for touch.

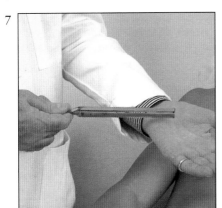

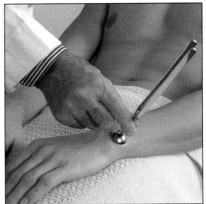

7 and 8 *Vibration* sense is assessed by applying the base of a clinical tuning fork to a bony prominence. The stimulus is generated by the examiner lightly tapping the fork on his/her hypothenar eminence. Strike the tuning fork before each application and ask the patient, with his eyes closed, whether the vibration is present and when it stops. Occasionally, deliberately stop the tuning fork to assess accuracy in response.

Start with wrist and ankle on each side, progress proximally to the olecranon and acrominion, and the patella and anterior superior iliac spine, if there is a distal absence.

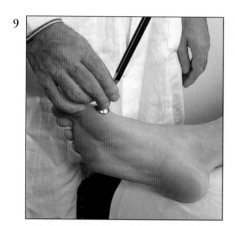

9 The feet are particularly important to assess in the diabetic patient for distal neuropathy.

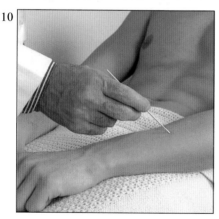

10 *Graphasthesia* is assessed by writing numbers or letters on each palm or forearm and the anterior compartment of each shin. Use a blunt object, such as the blunt end of a pen or pencil. With the patient's eyes closed, give examples for orientation and then assess: the numbers 3 and 8 are useful stimuli.

Assessment of size, shape and weight (stereognosis) is with common objects placed in the palm of the hand with the patient's eyes closed. Useful stimuli are coins, pens, pencils and keys. Check for deep pain sensation by squeezing the Achilles tendon from side to side or pressing the base of the thumb or great toenail.

11 Sensory inattention, typical of parietal lobe lesions, is elicited by the simultaneous application of stimuli on the two halves of the body. The patient has his eyes closed and occasionally only one side is touched.

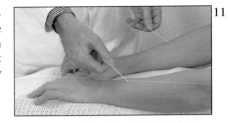

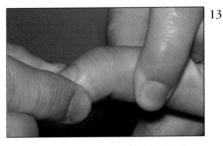

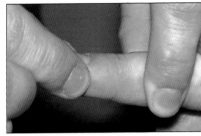

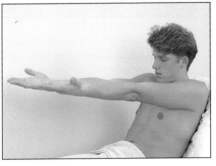

12 and 13 Joint *position sense* is examined in the upper and lower limbs starting distally and moving proximally if a defect is elicited. Hold the hand or foot with the left hand and with the right index finger and thumb gently grasp each side of the terminal phalanx of the index finger or great toe. Indicate to the patient up and down movements and then, with his eyes closed, ask him to identify a series of movements, inserting ups and downs in a random fashion. The normal subject will perceive minimal changes of angulation.

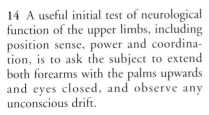

14 A useful initial test of neurological function of the upper limbs, including position sense, power and coordination, is to ask the subject to extend both forearms with the palms upwards and eyes closed, and observe any unconscious drift.

15 Romberg's sign is assessed by asking the patient to stand upright with feet together and eyes closed, the examiner guarding against any fall. An initial gentle sway of the body is normal but in abnormalities of dorsal column function, the subject is unable to stand unaided.

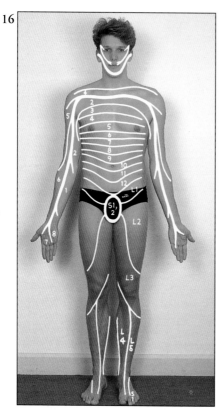

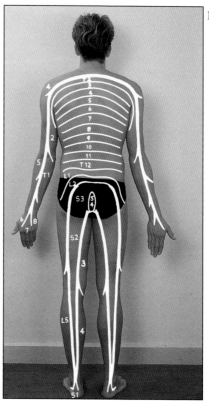

16 Anterior aspect of the body: cutaneous dermatomes: the bold lines indicate axial lines.

17 Posterior aspect of the body: cutaneous dermatomes: the bold lines indicate axial lines.

Motor Function

Examination of the motor system can be divided into assessment of tone, power, coordination, reflexes and abnormal movements. During this examination, one is also looking for wasting and other muscular abnormalities. Muscle abnormalities are considered in the following paragraphs, but may be indicative of musculoskeletal as well as neurological disease.

Muscle

Observe the symmetry and shape of muscles for evidence of hypertrophy, wasting, abnormal shape (e.g. torn tendons and contractures) and abnormal movement (p 179).

Palpation of muscles allows the assessment of *tone* and also identification and localisation of symptomatic and unsuspected tenderness. At some sites, peripheral nerves can be palpated for thickening and associated tenderness (e.g. the ulnar nerve behind the medial epicondyle of the humerus and the lateral popliteal nerve over the neck of the fibula).

Tapping along the course of a nerve may give an indication of sites of damage (over the median nerve at the wrist in carpal tunnel compression) or the level to which a regeneration has taken place after nerve transection (Tinnel's sign). Hypotonia may be present in muscle wasting disease (myotonia or peripheral nerve injuries) and hypertonia in established upper motor neurone disease.

The muscle bulk is related to age, sex, physical activity and to nutritional status. Atrophy may indicate primary muscle disease or peripheral nerve damage. The measure of the amount of wasting can be obtained with a tape measure, comparing the two limbs or repeated measurements after a timed interval. Measure the circumference at set distances from a bony landmark such as the tip of the shoulder in the upper arm, the olecranon for the forearm and the tibial tubercle for thigh and calf (p 186).

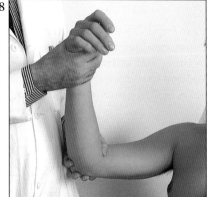

Tone

18 Tone is assessed in the upper and lower limbs by passive movement of the major joints. With the patient in a relaxed state, there should be minimal resistance to passive movement. Minor changes may be accentuated by requesting the subject to perform other activities simultaneously, such as moving the contralateral arm or leg and clenching their teeth.

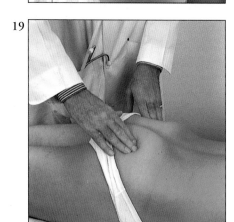

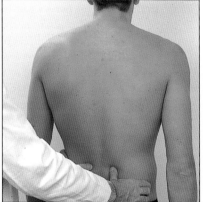

19 and 20 Palpating the bulk of muscles, such as the gluteus maximus or the erector spinae group, also provides information on their tone.

Power

Power is assessed by *active* movement of each joint in turn, comparing right with left and then adding *resistance* to these movements.

Passive Movement will locate joint pain and stiffness (p 184) and also identify contractures and assess tone, spasticity of upper motor neurone lesions and the clasp-like cog wheel rigidity of diseases of the basal ganglia.

Assessment of power of active movement begins with observation of posture and gait. It is then specifically determined by movements of each joint and individual muscle, by testing specific movements while eliminating the action of accessory muscles and tricks which overcome any individual muscle weakness. When assessing this power an indication is also obtained of the control of antagonistic muscles, the smoothness and coordination of movements and whether they are being limited by pain, contractures or joint abnormalities.

Initially gross movements are used to compare the limbs, such as hand shaking, flexion and extension of joints. Power can be graded from 0 to 5: 0, no contracture; 1, a flicker of movement; 2, active movement with gravity excluded; 3, active against gravity; 4, active against gravity and resistance (plus and minus signs are used to divide this group); 5, normal.

Resisted Movements of Individual Muscles and Muscle Groups

21 A measure of the power of spinal flexion can be obtained by asking the subject to raise his head and shoulders off the couch while supporting his thighs. Resistance can be added by pressure applied to the sternum. In resisted movements, the subject is asked to prevent the examiner from moving the part away from a fixed position.

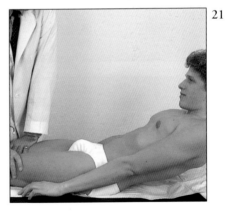

21

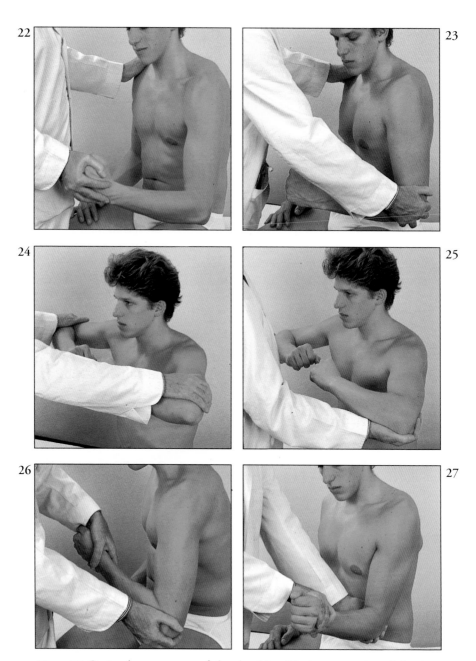

22 to 27 Resisted movements of the shoulder. Flexion, extension abduction, adduction, internal rotation and external rotation.

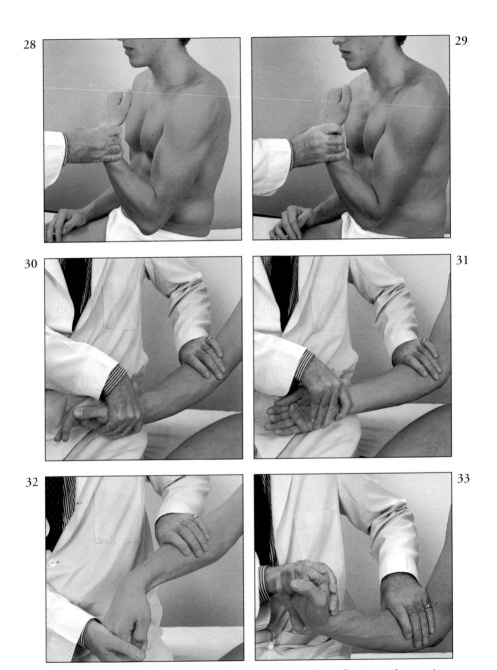

28 to 33 Resisted movements of elbow and wrist: elbow flexion and extension, pronation, supination, wrist flexion and extension.

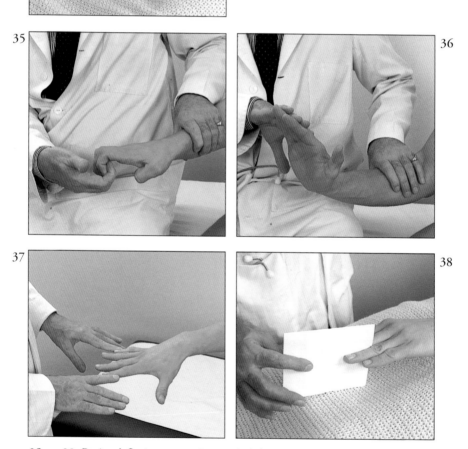

34 Comparing hand grips.

35 to 38 Resisted flexion, extension and abduction, gripping by adduction of the fingers.

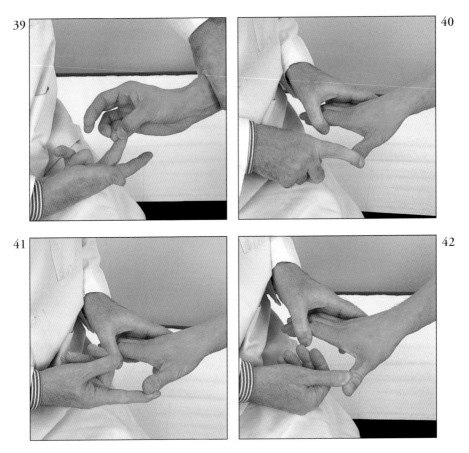

39 to 42 Resisted opposition, extension, abduction and adduction of the thumb.

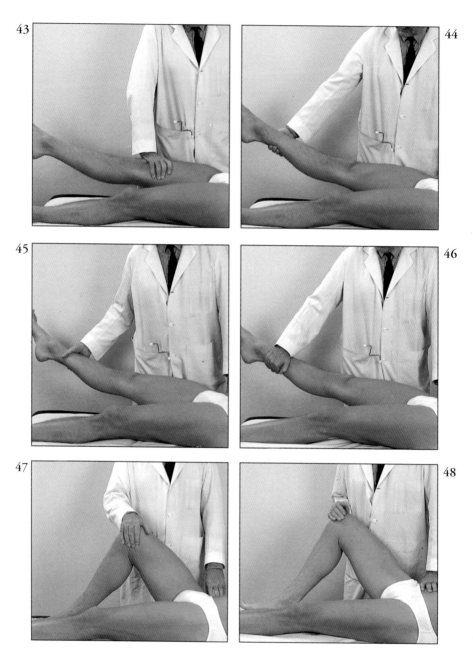

43 to 48 Resisted movements of the hip joint: flexion, extension, abduction, adduction, internal rotation and external rotation.

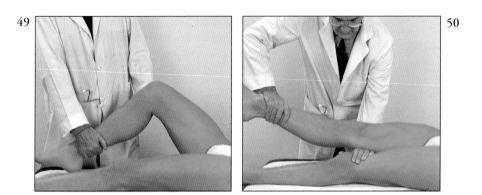

49 and 50 Resisted flexion and extension of the knee.

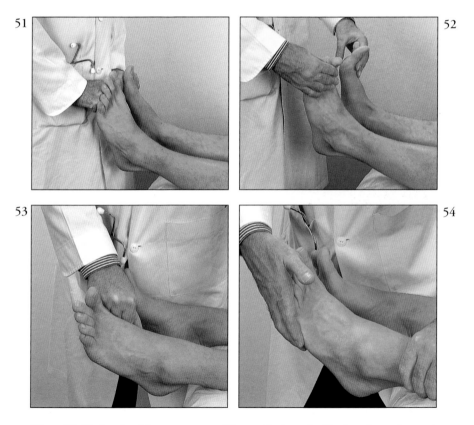

51 to 54 Resisted ankle movements. Plantar flexion, doriflexion, inversion and eversion.

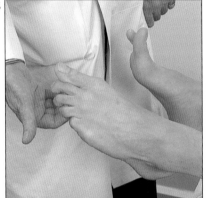

55 to 57 Resisted toe movements. Flexion, extension and abduction. The power of dorsiflexion of the great toe is a useful test of the L5 nerve root, since this is not involved in lower limb reflex innervation (p 176).

56

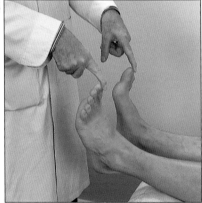

57

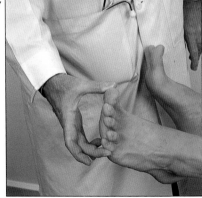

Coordination

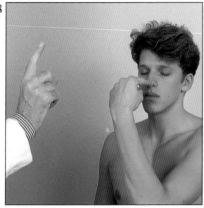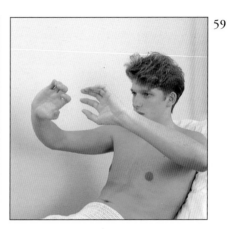

58 and 59 Coordination of upper limb movements is assessed by alternatively touching an examiner's finger and the subject's nose. The examiner moves the finger from side to side or leaves it in position and asks the patient to repeat the movement with closed eyes. The patient is also asked to describe circles and figures with the outstretched arm, or screw up imaginary jam jars.

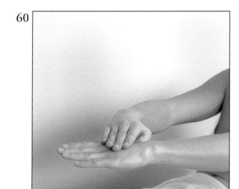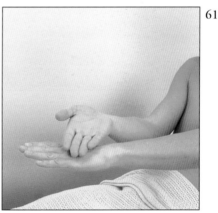

60 and 61 Fine movements can be assessed by tapping the dorsum of the contralateral hand alternatively with the front and back of the fingers.

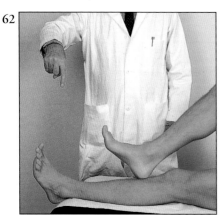

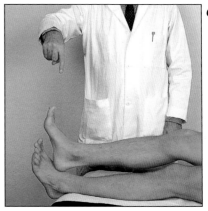

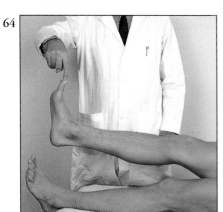

62 to 64 In the lower limb each heel can be placed in turn on the contralateral shin and moved from knee to ankle and back, or from knee to ankle and on to a strategically placed finger.

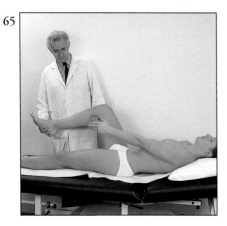

65 Also, describing circles with the great toe or, with closed eyes, to 'shoot' the passively moved foot with two fingers.

172

66 Disturbances of gait can be accentuated by asking the subject to walk in a straight line and repeat this heel to toe fashion. Ataxia (incoordination of gait) may be due to altered state of consciousness (e.g. excess alcohol, head injury, upper motor neurone spasticity), altered tone of cerebellar and basal ganglia disease and abnormalities of sensory input, where the subject is unaware of the position in space.

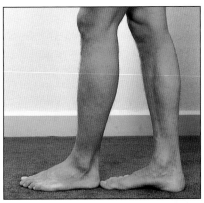

66

Assess the subject standing still, feet together and eyes closed, when abnormalities of posture may be accentuated (p 159, Romberg's sign).

67

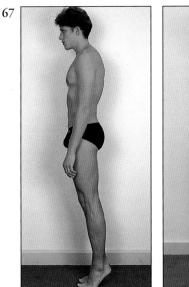

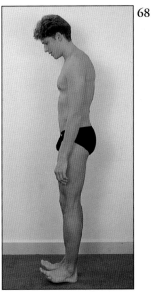

68

67 and 68 Standing on toes and heels are further tests of coordination, but also depend on position sense, muscle power and normal joints. The altered coordination of cerebellar disease is characteristically slow, awkward and incomplete, requiring a few tries to complete a movement and is termed dysdiadochokinesis.

Reflexes

Assessment of *deep* and *superficial reflexes* provides information on the integrity of reflex arcs at different levels in the central nervous system. They may be abolished by disease of the lower motor neurone or sensory neurones in the reflex arc and may be modified by central damage, such as in hyper-reflexic upper motor neurone lesions.

When testing limb reflexes, the position of the limb is such as to put slight tension on the stimulated muscle, but supporting the weight to avoid any active tension. Appropriate tendons are struck precisely and gently with a patellar hammer from a few centimetres swing. Sluggish reflexes can be reinforced by requesting the subject to clench his teeth or pull opposing clasped fingers.

69 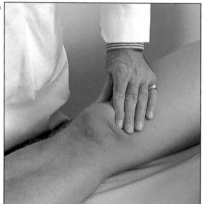 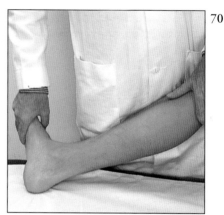 70

69 and 70 In hyper-reflexia, stimulation of one muscle may produce movements elsewhere, e.g. antagonists or more distant muscle. In marked hyper-reflexia, tension on the muscle alone may produce reflex contraction, or sustained tension repeated jerking movement (clonus), as demonstrated by patellar and ankle clonus.

If the stimulated muscle is weak the stimulus may produce movement in powerful antagonist muscles (paradoxical or inverted reflexes). Hyporeflexia may persist after motor nerve recovery in a peripheral nerve injury but is not a good indicator of the severity of the lesion. Reflexes may persist until late in the course of muscular disease.

Reflexes may be graded by the degree of contraction: 0, not elicited; 1, elicited with reinforcement; 2, normal; 3, brisk; 4 and 5, unsustained and sustained clonus.

Specific reflex nerve root levels are: biceps, C5,6; supinator and triceps, C6,7; Knee, L3,4; Ankle, S1,2.

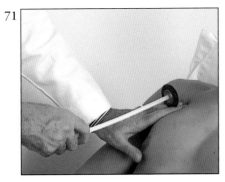

71 Pectoralis major reflex.

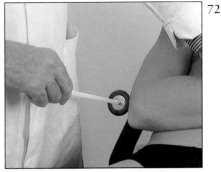

72 Triceps reflex.

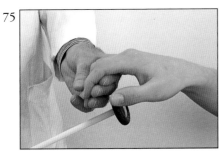

73 Biceps reflex.

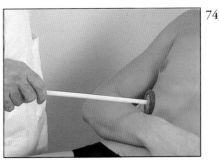

74 Supinator reflex.

75 Finger jerk.

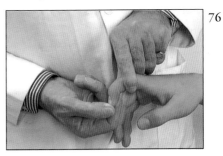

76 Hoffman reflex.

77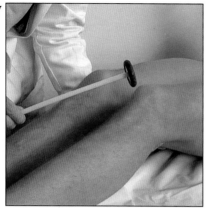

77 Knee jerk.

78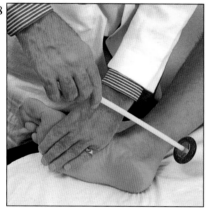

78 and 79 Ankle jerk.

79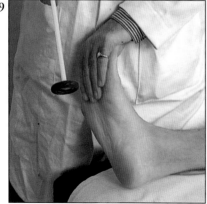

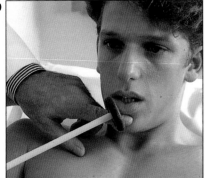

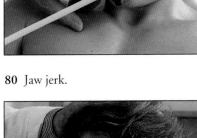

80 Jaw jerk.

81 Oroangular reflex.

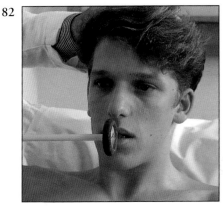

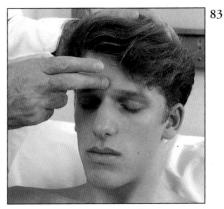

82 Pouting reflex.

83 Glabellar tap.

84 Of the superficial responses, the Babinski is routinely examined. It is elicited by scratching the outer edge of the sole from the heel forwards with a key or other implement, a normal response being curling downwards of the toes. A positive (abnormal) Babinski response is extension and fanning of the toes; this is present at birth but, after this time, is indicative of an upper motor neurone lesion.

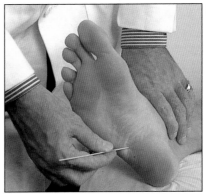

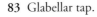

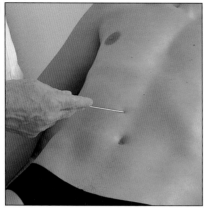

 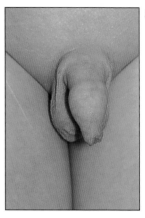

86

85 Abdominal reflexes are elicited by scratching diagonally across the four quadrants, each producing contraction of the underlying abdominal musculature.

86 The cremasteric reflex is contraction of the cremaster muscle on one side, by stroking the adjacent upper inner thigh. (Note the scratch mark on the inner thigh and the contracted cremaster muscle on this side.)

 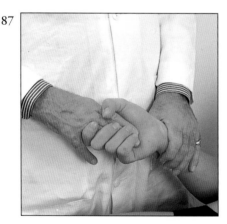

 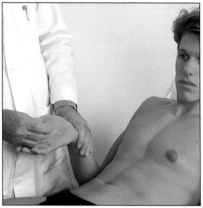

87 Some reflexes are most prominent at birth. These are the grasp reflex, produced by stroking the palm, and the placing reaction of the sole, produced by touching the outer border of the dependent foot.

88 The palmo-mental reflex is the movement of the angle of the mouth on scratching the ipsilateral hypothenar eminence.

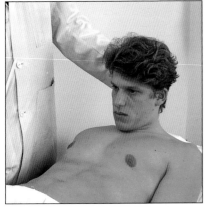 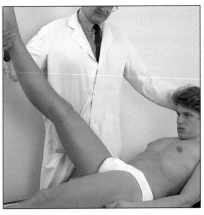

89 and 90   At the end of motor system examination check for neck rigidity (Kernig's sign) by raising the patient's head off the bed. Neck stiffness can also be elicited by simultaneous neck and straight leg raising or by bending the hip to a right angle with bent knee and then straightening the leg in this position.

Abnormal Movements

Abnormal movements include epilepsy, tremors (e.g. Parkinson's disease), spasm, the clonus of upper motor neurone disturbance, and the athetoid and choreiform movements of birth injuries and chorea. Fascicular movements (flickering) of muscles occur in motor neurone disease and may indicate a hyperexcitable muscle, the movement being produced by gentle tapping.

In summary, upper motor neurone lesions initially produce paralysis and hypotonia but subsequently develop weakness, spasticity, hyper-reflexia and an extensor plantar response. Extra-pyramidal lesions interfere with the balance of muscle activity, affecting tone, coordination and involuntary movement, without marked loss of power. Cerebellar lesions produce hypotonia and ataxia; lower motor neurone lesions produce weakness, wasting, hypotonia and areflexia.

Autonomic Nervous System

Denervation of the sympathetic supply of the limb produces vasodilatation and loss of sweating. Initially there is rosy colouring of the digits but this may progress to mottling, oedema and lowering of the temperature. Degenerative (trophic) changes may develop, giving smooth skin and some spindling due to pulp atrophy. Hyperkeratinisation may develop on traumatised areas, together with loss of hair, trauma lines across the nails and clubbing.

Cranial nerve autonomic changes include defects of lacrimation, salivation, swallowing and gut motility. Pupillary reflexes may be lost, as will the normal heart rate changes with respiration (sinus arrhythmia), hyperventilation (30 breaths per minute for 20 seconds should raise the heart rate by 12 beats per minute), Valsalva (reduction heart rate), carotid sinus massage (reduction of heart rate), postural change from lying to standing (a rise of 20–30 beats per minute). The latter reflex reduces blood pressure fall, but this may be up to 10mm of mercury in a normal elderly person. Abnormalities of the sacral parasympathetic innervation include altered tone in the anal and urinary sphincters.

Checklist for the Assessment of the Nervous System

History

Current mental state: level of consciousness; orientation; memory; intellect; understanding; insight; thought content; behaviour; mood; hallucinations; delusions.

Headache; fits, faints, falls; dizziness.

Disturbances of vision/speech; Diplopia, visual loss; dysarthria, dysphasia.

Disturbances of motor or sensory function of limbs/face: dysaesthesia, clumsiness, weakness.

Examination

Handedness; NB compare the two sides of the body.

Speech: dysphasia (expressive, receptive, global), jargon, scanning, stuttering; dysarthria.

Cranial Nerves

I—smell

II—visual acuity; visual fields; fundoscopy

III, IV, VI—pupillary responses to light and accommodation; enophthalmus; exophthalmos; ptosis; lid lag; nystagmus; extra-ocular movements

V—sensation over the three nerve divisions; corneal reflex; muscles of mastication, jaw jerk

VII—facial expression; taste anterior ⅔ tongue

VIII—hearing; Rinne's and Weber's tests

IX—gag reflex; taste posterior ⅓ tongue

X—voice; cough; uvular deviation

XI—shoulder shrugging, neck rotation

XII—tongue movements

Motor Function

Tone: spasticity, flaccidity, rigidity; clonus

Power: hand grips, wrists, elbows, shoulder, ankles, knees, hips

Coordination: finger–nose, heel–shin; dysdiadochokinesis; pyramidal drift

Reflexes: tendon, superficial

Abnormal movements: tremor (static, intention); choreiform; athetoid; convulsions; associated movements; tics

Muscle: wasting; hypertrophy; fasciculation

Abnormalities of posture: upper/lower motor neurone; extrapyramidal; cerebellar; sensory; myopathic; Romberg's sign

Gait: (NB walking must be assessed) spastic; ataxic; waddling; limp

Sensory—nerve root, spinal cord level, hemianaesthesia

Light touch: cotton wool

Pain: pinprick

Temperature: finger/tuning fork

Position sense: hold sides of digits

Vibration: start distally on wrist and ankle

Graphasthesia: use threes and eights

Two-point discrimination: blunt compass, start on hand

Stereognosis: coins, keys

Autonomic

Sweating; postural hypotension; heart rate response to a Valsalva manoeuvre

Spinal deformity/tenderness; neck rigidity

Palpate and percuss abnormal superficial nerves

Contractures: neuropathic joints; ulceration

Carotid bruits

The Musculoskeletal System

The musculo-skeletal system comprises the joints, bones and muscles. This section considers the general and individual examination of the *joints* and their adjacent *bones; muscular* assessment is considered in more detail with the nervous system (p 161).

Bones and Joints

Formal examination of every joint does not form part of a routine physical examination. More often it is directed by a patient's history and abnormalities noted on general inspection. All students must, however, learn how to examine each joint: the principles are to *look, feel, move, measure* and *x-ray.*

Inspection (Look)

A patient must be appropriately undressed; always compare right with left, and with abnormalities of other joints. Note *skin,* colour, rashes, creases, scars, sinuses and contractures. Erythema may indicate arthritis or infection, while a rash may give important clues to underlying joint disturbances. Abnormal *shape* of a joint may reflect swelling due to effusions, synovial hypertrophy, inflammation and bony overgrowths.

Deformity may be postural (due to abnormal posture) or structural (due to tissue abnormalities), paralytic (due to muscular imbalance) or compensatory (to overcome abnormalities elsewhere). The deformity may be mobile or fixed, i.e. not changeable on passive movement: the deformities may be symmetrical or asymmetrical. The degree of deformity may be mild (e.g. ulnar deviation of the metacarpophalangeal joint in early rheumatoid arthritis) or gross (e.g. destruction of a denervated joint in a neuropathic disturbance).

Lateral deviation of the distal portion of a joint in relation to the proximal is termed a valgus, and medial deviation a varus, deformity. Abnormalities of bone alignment are classified as subluxation, when the displaced parts of joint surfaces remain in contact, and dislocation when there is loss of contact between the two adjacent surfaces.

The observer should note any alteration in the shape or outline of the bone, localized swelling and evidence of tenderness. Bones may be both deformed and enlarged, as in osteitis deformans (Paget's disease), or there may be alteration of their shape, as in the bowing of the tibia seen in rickets.

Atrophy of muscles may suggest disuse, injury, myopathy or neuropathy and abnormal movements should be noted. Tendons and bursae are examined for inflammatory changes.

Palpation (Feel)

Palpation of the joint should detect *warmth* which may signify an active synovitis or infection and *tenderness* of the joint or periarticular tissues. Stroking a limb from proximal to distal encounters a gradual cooling of temperature and abnormality can be readily appreciated. The history will indicate the presence of painful sites and the examiner must show extreme gentleness; watch a patient's face during palpation, and later in active and passive movement. Tenderness is an important sign of pathology, localize its site as accurately as possible. Remember, however, that tenderness, like pain, can be referred from a damaged to a distant area.

The joint is systematically palpated for evidence of *swelling*: this may be of the skin, subcutaneous tissues, muscles, joint capsule, synovial membrane, bone or intracapsular structures, such as an effusion or abnormal cartiliges. Synovial thickening and synovitis have a soft and boggy characteristic. An effusion is fluctuant and fluid can be made to shift within the joint. Any altered cutaneous sensation is mapped out.

Tenderness of bones is characteristic of osteitis fibrosa, multiple myeloma, leukaemic infiltration of bones, secondary deposits and osteomyelitis. Fractures may be accompanied by swelling, deformity, crepitus, abnormal mobility and loss of function.

Movement

In examining movement of a joint it is important to first ask the patient specifically about pain and tenderness in the joint or the limb being examined. Initially the range of *active* movements is tested *before* proceeding to a more thorough evaluation of *passive* movement. Asking a patient to demonstrate the full range of active movement reveals the extent of dysfunction of a joint. For example asking the patient to do up a shirt button may reveal the extent of dysfunction of a hand.

Movement of a damaged muscle or its tendons commonly produce pain. This pain can be demonstrated by the examiner holding a joint in the mid range of a muscle activity, while the patient forcibly contracts this muscle. As no movement takes place, any pain can be localized to a specific muscle rather than the rigid elements or other muscles acting on the joint. In this 'resisted movement technique' (p 163), the examiner requires knowledge of the action of each muscle in order to stand in the appropriate position to hold and resist activity. Note is also taken of any muscle weakness. Power (p 163) is graded on a scale of 0 to 5: 5 being normal and 0 total paralysis.

Passive movement must be executed with extreme gentleness and a patient's face watched during the maneouvres. These precautions will give the patient confidence to totally relax while the examiner tests the full range of movement in each joint. The commonest cause of limited movement is pain of the structures attached to the joint or elsewhere within the limb. It may be due to inflammatory changes. Other causes are thickening of the capsule and periarticular structures, joint effusions, muscle spasm or contractures and bony irregularities or ankyloses. Excessive movement in unstable joints may be due to lax or torn ligaments and bony deformity. A grating or creaking sensation, *crepitus*, may be felt across a joint, suggesting irregularity of the articular cartilaginous surfaces.

Movement involves both the neurological and musculoskeletal systems, the emphasis in the former being on tone, power, coordination and reflexes, while in the latter the emphasis is on the measurement of active and passive movement. There is, however, a considerable overlap. In this text, to avoid excessive repetition, the neurological examination considers muscle abnormalities (p 161) and the power of movement, while in this chapter, the normal extent of active and passive movement are emphasized. In practice the student will need to master all techniques for assessing active, passive and resisted movement, and muscle power for use in either system.

Measurement

1 Measurement of joint movement requires the use of a goniometer which is a hinged rod with a protractor at its centre. This allows the jaws to be opened and aligned with the bones on either side. Movement may thus be recorded as the number of degrees in each direction, compared with the normal and that of the other side, indicating abnormalities of range and deformity. It is unusual for the goniometer to be used by non-rheumatologists and most clinicians merely estimate these joint angles.

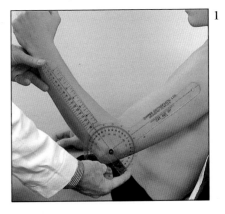

1

2

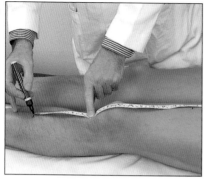

3

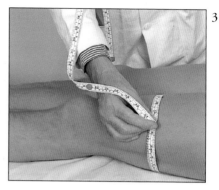

2 and 3 A tape measure is used to measure the circumference of limbs at fixed sites, to determine evidence of muscle wasting. In the lower limb, palpate the upper prominence of the tibial tubercle and use this fixed point for measurement. In the adult male, 25cm proximal and 10cm distal to this point provide useful markers but choose the most appropriate measures to match muscle bulk.

Be sure to use the same markers on each side, and record the distance and the circumference in the patient's notes.

4

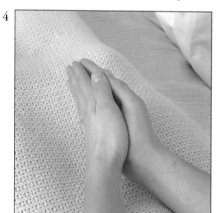

5

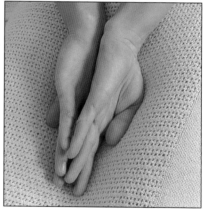

4 and 5 Muscle bulk can be compared directly between the two sides of the body, as with the thenar and hypothenar eminences.

Measurement of the length of the whole or part of each limb establishes real or apparent shortening (p 213). The various segments are measured not only in developmental assessment (p 32), but also to demonstrate shortening due to congenital abnormalities or injuries.

Spine

Inspection

The spine is initially examined in the standing position with the hands relaxed at each side. The entire posterior aspect of the trunk should be exposed, the subject wearing small briefs and being barefooted. Observe the posture from behind and from each side. Note the natural cervical, thoracic and lumbar curvatures. The thoracic curvature may be more pronounced with increased age, abnormal prominence is termed kyphosis. The lumbar curve is more marked in females and excessive curvature is termed lordosis.

Bony landmarks are the spinus processes, the angles of the scapulae, the ribs, and the crests and posterior superior iliac spines of the pelvis. A shallow pit (Dimple of Venus) may be present over each sacroiliac joint in the female. The spines should be in the midline and the two sides of the body symmetrical. The vertebra prominens is the spine of C7. Note any steps in the spinous processes, indicating abnormalities of the underlying vertebra.

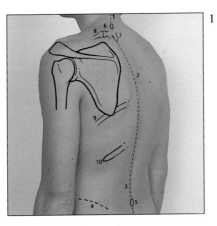

1 Spinal curvatures

1	Cervical curvature	8	First rib
2	Dorsal curvature	9	Seventh rib
3	Lumbar curvature	10	Twelfth rib
4	Superior iliac crest		
5	Spinous process of 4th lumbar vertebra		
6	Spinous process of 7th cervical vertebra		
7	Spinous process of 1st thoracic vertebra		

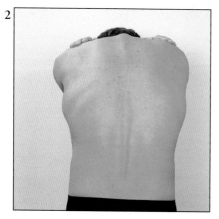

2 Deviation of the spines from the midline is termed scoliosis. This may be mild and postural in nature, and can be overcome by asking the subject to place each hand on the opposite shoulder and to lean forward. The latter movement will accentuate a pathological scoliosis. Scoliosis is accompanied by rotation of the bodies of the vertebra so that the spines point to the cavity of the curve. Kyphosis and scoliosis are thus often combined.

Palpation

Before commencing to palpate, ask the patient to point out any site of discomfort. It may be appropriate to mark this site to direct attention in the examination and ensure consistency of the witness.

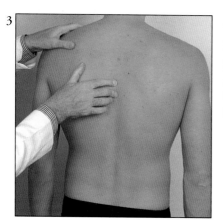

3 The spines can be felt in a thin subject from C6 down to the sacrum and the tip of the index finger inserted between them to locate any tender spots. Palpation is also undertaken along either side, over the transverse processes and the intervertebral joints.

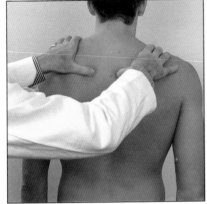

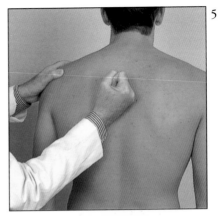

4 to 6 If no tenderness is elicited, pressure can be increased by using both thumbs, digital percussion or tapping the spine with a fist or tapping a fist on the other hand.

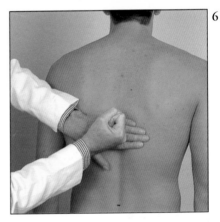

Altered sensation on either side of the midline can be demonstrated by simultaneous digital dragging or pinching the skin on each side. Palpation of the muscles on either side, particularly in the lumbar region, will assess the presence of spasm: lumbar spasm may also be accompanied by loss of the normal lumbar lordosis (p 187).

7

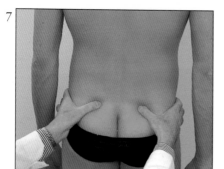

7 The sacroiliac joints are subcutaneous and palpable for areas of tenderness.

Movement

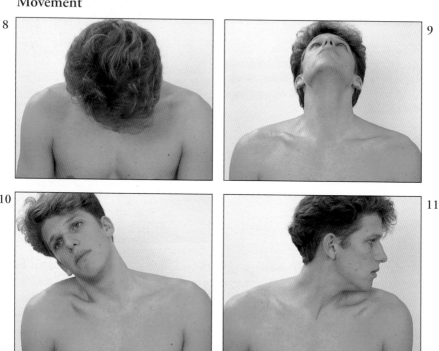

8 to 11 Active and passive movements of the cervical spine are usually assessed independently of the rest of the back. Flexion is tested by asking the patient to put his chin on his chest (normal 45 degrees) and extension by looking upwards and backwards (45 degrees). Lateral flexion is by approximating the ear to the adjacent shoulder on each side and is approximately 45 degrees. Rotation is by looking over each shoulder and is normally 75 degrees.

12 Much of the apparent flexion on leaning forward to touch one's toes, with straight legs, takes place at the atlanto-occipital and hip joints. In the cervical region flexion straightens the cervical curve. There is little movement in the thoracic spine but flexion is maximum in the lumbar region. The distance of the finger tips from the ground on bending forward varies with age and between individuals. It can also be used to monitor progress of any limitation of movement and of the point of onset of pain.

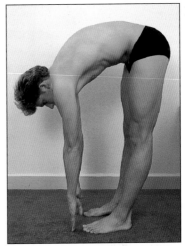

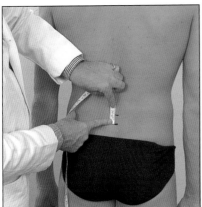 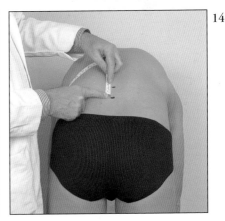

13 and 14 The spines can be marked and the distances between any chosen levels measured with a tape measure before and after flexion.

15

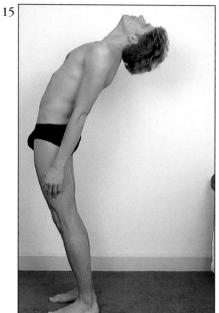

16

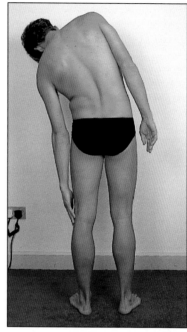

17

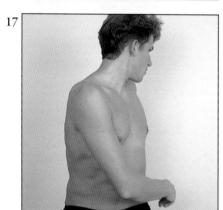

15 to 17 Extension is assessed by leaning backwards. Lateral flexion is assessed when the patient slides a hand down each thigh in turn. Rotation can be masked by pelvic movement and the pelvis has to be fixed by the examiner's hands while turning the head and shoulders maximally to each side or, more conveniently, with the patient sitting down.

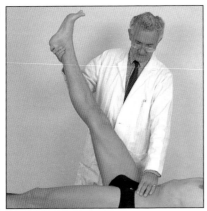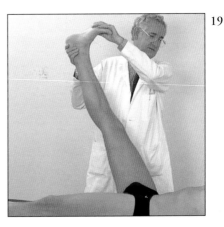

19

18 and 19 Limitation of straight leg raising, lifting the patient's heel, indicates tension on the radicles of the sciatic nerve and may be indicative of lumbar disc abnormalities. The sign may be accentuated by simultaneous dorsiflexion of the ankle.

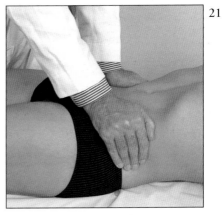

20 and 21 The integrity of the pelvis is examined by side to side compression on the iliac bones, pressure on the pubis in the sagittal plane, and simultaneous backward pressure on the two iliac crests.

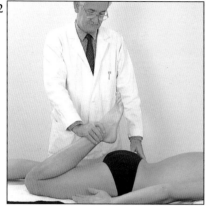

22 Further assessment is with the patient lying prone. Tension is applied to the femoral nerve by passively flexing each knee in turn. Pressure is applied over the sacrum to identify pelvic pain.

Other essential components of the examination of back pain, are a neurological assessment, and a rectal and/or vaginal examination to ensure that pathology within the pelvis is not causing the symptom.

Regional Examination of the Joints

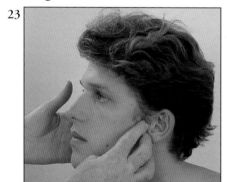
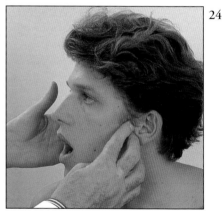

23 and 24 The temporomandibular joint is subcutaneous and palpable laterally. The condyle can be felt to glide over the zygomatic tubercle on opening the mouth. The muscles of mastication are considered on p 149. The joint may click, dislocate, or be involved in arthritic changes.

Upper Limb

The initial application of a few simple tests may serve to localize upper limb abnormalities. These may for example include picking up objects, writing, asking the patient to put his hands together, as if praying, or to comb his hair. Functional limitation and sites of the problem thus usually become apparent. A full regional examination is then performed involving inspection, palpation and movement of all joints and periarticular structures. Assessment of muscle power, and neurological function should also be carried out.

Shoulder Girdle

Shoulder movements are composite, involving the ball and socket articulation at the shoulder (glenohumeral) joint, together with movements between the scapula and clavicle, and the thorax.

Inspection

Swelling of the shoulder joint may be visible due to joint effusion, or synovial thickening. Deformity of the joint, and dislocation may be apparent.

Palpation

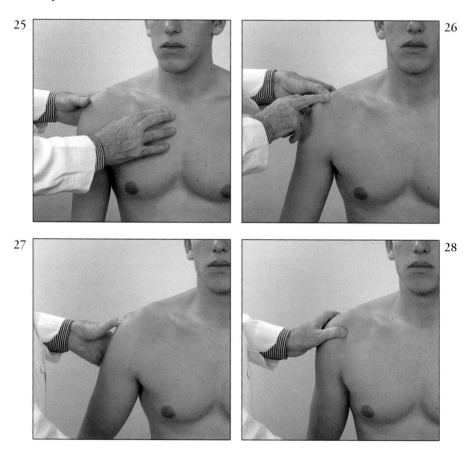

25 to 28 Palpation of the sternoclavicular joint, acromioclavicular joint, subacromial bursa and the head of the humerus.

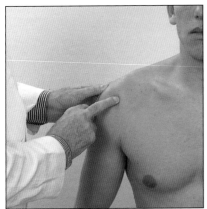 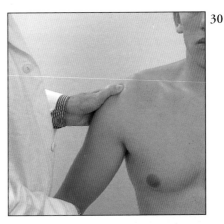

29 and 30 The greater and lesser tuberosities are separated by the bicipital groove containing the long tendon of the biceps muscle and its bursa.

Movement

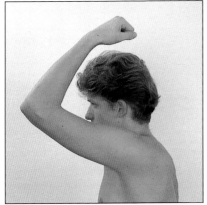 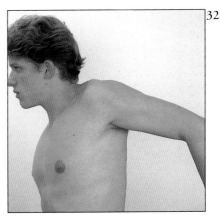

31 and 32 The shoulder joint allows flexion, extension, abduction, adduction, external and internal rotation, and circumduction. Flexion is possible to 180 degrees, the arm being swung forward as in marching: this involves some scapula movement, the glenohumeral joint contributing about 90 degrees. Extension at the shoulder is possible to 65 degrees, the arm being swung backward.

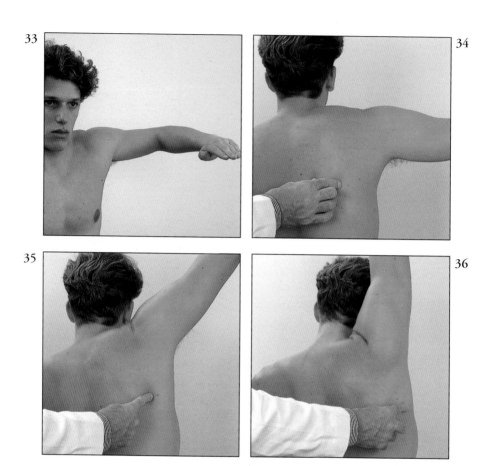

33 to 36 Arm abduction takes place at both the glenohumeral joint and through scapular rotation. On its own (assessed by fixing the scapula) the former is to 90 degrees. When the movement of the scapula is included, 180 degrees is possible. However, there also has to be external rotation of the shoulder joint for the greater tuberosity to clear the acromion.

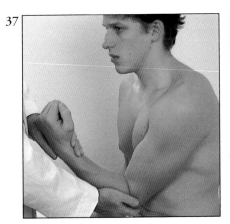

37

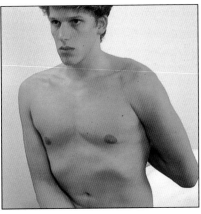

38

37 Adduction is possible to 50 degrees in the normal joint, the arm being carried forward across the front of the chest.

38 Internal rotation is possible to 90 degrees, the patient being asked to scratch his back with the thumb as high as possible.

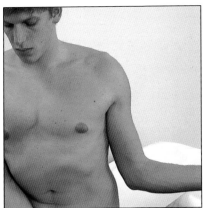

39

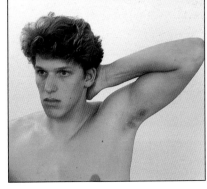

40

39 and 40 External rotation is to 60 degrees and is assessed with a flexed elbow. Placing the hand behind the head incorporates abduction and external rotation.

Elbow and Radio-Ulnar Joints

Inspect for joint effusion or swellings, and discrete swellings over the olecranon or over the proximal subcutaneous border of the ulnar (e.g. rheumatoid nodules, gouty tophi, tuberous xanthomas).

41

42

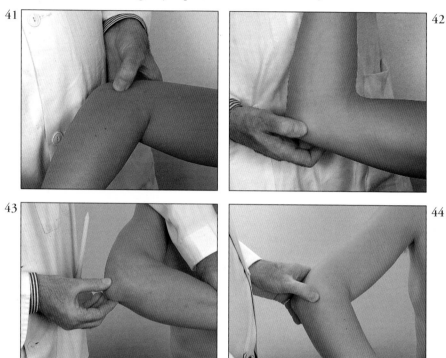

43

44

45

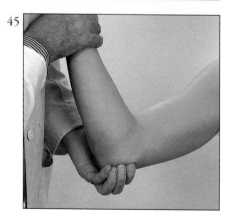

41 to 45   A number of the bony components of the elbow and superior radio-ulnar joints are palpable. These include the lateral and medial epicondyles, the olecranon and the head of the radius. The ulnar nerve can be palpated behind the medial epicondyle.

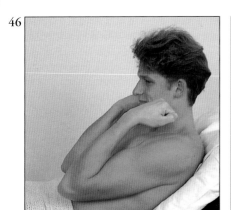

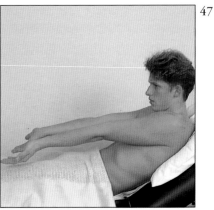

46 and 47 The elbow joint is a hinge joint, and the zero position is when the arm is fully extended (zero degrees) normal flexion being possible to approximately 150 degrees. Early synovitis may limit extension.

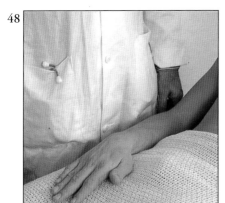

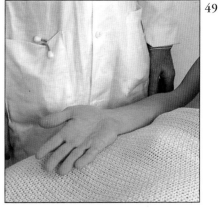

48 and 49 With the elbow flexed to 90 degrees, pronation and supination may be tested. About 80 degrees supination and 80 degrees pronation are possible. Pronation and supination take place at both the superior and inferior radio- ulnar joints.

50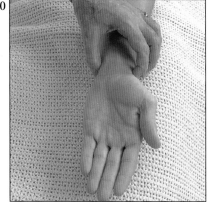

50 Note that in full supination (in the anatomical position with the palm facing forwards) the radial and ulnar styloid processess can be palpated, the radial styloid being approximately 1cm distal to the ulnar. This is an important relationship, since fractures of the lower end of the radius are common and impaction displaces the radial styloid proximally, and the two styloid processess often end up at the same level.

51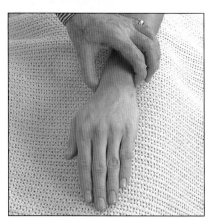

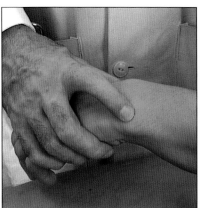 52

51 and 52 During pronation the radial styloid is still palpable but on the other side of the wrist it is the head, and not the styloid process, of the ulnar which can be palpated.

Wrist and Hand

Wrist Joint

53 Inspect the wrist for erythema, swelling, deformity and muscle wasting. The wrist is palpated with both thumbs placed on the dorsal surface, with the wrist supported underneath with the index fingers. A boggy swelling may signify the presence of synovitis or effusions.

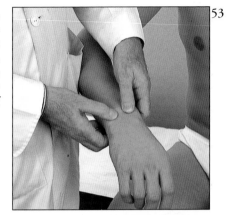
53

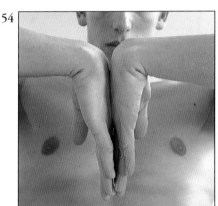
54

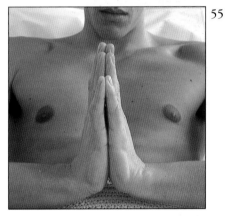
55

54 and 55 Flexion is examined by asking the patient to approximate the dorsum of his hands together and flex the wrist joint: it should be approximately 90 degrees. The patient is asked to put both hands together and then extend the forearms. Extension at this joint should be 85–90 degrees.

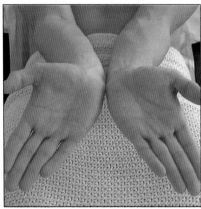
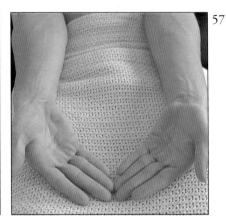

57

56 and 57 Radial and ulnar deviation at the wrist sould be about 20 degrees and 50 degrees respectively. Similar ranges should be achieved in active and passive movements.

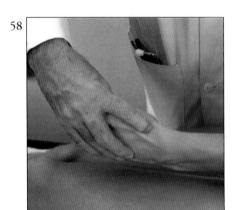

58 Palpating proximally to distally in the anatomical snuff box are the radial styloid, the wrist joint margin and the scaphoid bone. Fractures of the latter can be easily missed and an important physical sign is tenderness of the bone at this site.

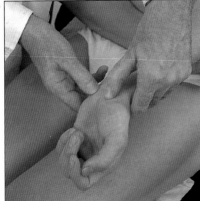
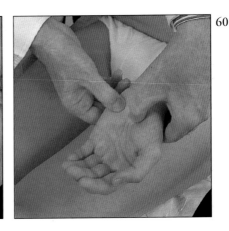

59 and 60 The flexor retinaculum is attached to four palpable bony structures and is only the size of a postage stamp. It has important clinical implications as the median nerve can be compressed beneath it, particularly after injury or with arthritic changes to the wrist or carpus. The bony attachments are proximally the tubercle of the scaphoid, and the pisiform bone, and distally the ridge of the trapezium and the hook of the hammate.

Metacarpophalangeal Joints

61

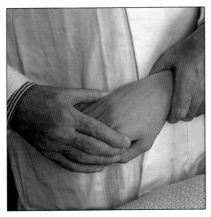
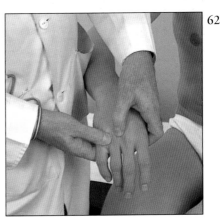

62

61 and 62 Lateral and antero-posterior pressure over the metacarpophalangeal joints is applied to elicit tenderness; this may be an early sign of inflammatory disease. Flexion of the straight fingers is to 90 degrees. The capacity to hyperextend should be noted and such hypermobility of joints may suggest underlying Marfan's or Ehlers-Danlos syndrome.

Interphalangeal Joints

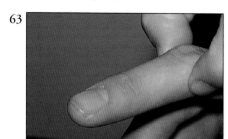

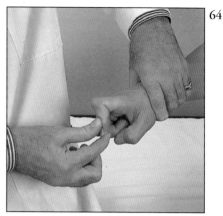

63 and 64 The sides of the interphalangeal joints are subcutaneous and can be palpated for local tenderness. There should be no hyperextension at the proximal interphalangeal joint; flexion is to 120 degrees if the distal interphalangeal joint is kept fully extended.

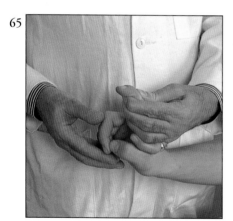

65 Flexion of the distal interphalangeal joint is approximately 80 degrees.

The Hand

The patient's fingers are passively flexed and extended while the examiner's fingers are palpating the flexor tendons to detect crepitus or restriction of movement from tenosynovitis. Power of the interossei muscles is assessed by asking the patient to keep the fingers spread apart against resistance (p 166).

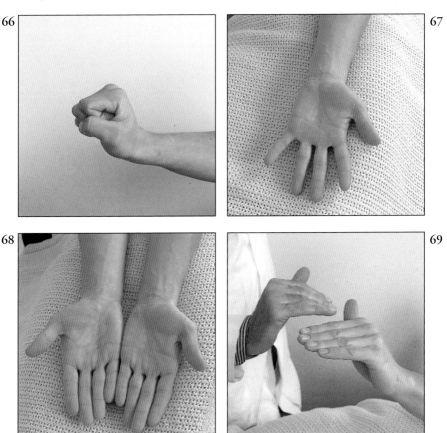

66 to 69 Useful composite movements to assess locomotor function of the hand are to make a fist, abduct and adduct the fingers and to flex the metacarpalpalangeal joints to a right angle with extended interphalangeal joints. The latter movement is produced by the lumbrical muscles with synergistic activity of the long flexor and extensor tendons.

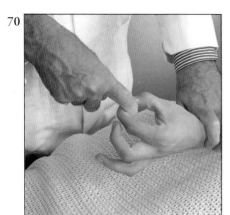

70

70 Opposition can be tested by trying to force apart the opposed thumb and little finger. A more practical approach is to ask the patient to undo a button, or write with a pen. Individual hand movements are further considered in the neurological section (p 166).

Lower Limb

Hip Joint

Inspection and Palpation

Initial assessment of the hip joint is with the patient lying flat and straight on a couch, in the supine position, with a single head pillow and wearing briefs. The neutral position of the hip is in extension with the patella pointing forward. Although the muscles and bones around the joint limit the value of inspection and palpation, an abnormal posture of the limb may indicate pain, deformity and altered mobility. Symmetry of skin creases and the contour of the thighs and buttocks are observed in each part of the examination. The anterior surface marking of the joint is just inferior and posterior to the mid-inguinal point and pressure at this site may reveal joint tenderness.

The greater trochanter is palpable and is on or just below a line joining the anterior superior iliac spine with the ischial tuberosity (Nelaton's line).

The intersection point of the line passing vertically backwards onto the couch through the anterior superior iliac spine and the horizontal line through the greater trochanter, is approximately 4cm from the trochanter in the adult. Reduction of this distance may indicate abnormalities of the neck of the femur. The triangle of this intersection point and the two bony markings make up Bryant's triangle.

1 Lateral aspect of the hip joint

1 Anterior superior iliac spine
2 Cranial limit of greater trochanter
3 Bryant's triangle. The distance B–C is shortened in fractures of the neck of the femur, this being demonstrated by comparing the distance B–C on the two sides.

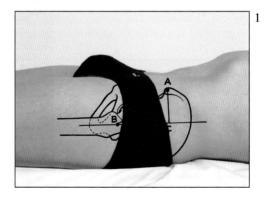

1

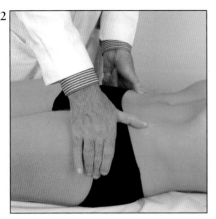

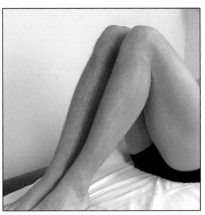

2 The relative position of the two hip joints can be roughly compared by placing thumbs on the anterior superior iliac spines and middle fingers on the greater trochanters.

3 If both knees are bent and the feet placed together on the couch, differences in leg length may be demonstrated by differences in the position of the two knee joints.

Movement and Measurement

Abnormalities of hip movement can be masked by compensatory movement of the pelvis and various manoevures are thus required to distinguish between the two components. Active and passive movements in each direction are examined concurrently to avoid doubly positioning the patient. The ipsilateral hand is used to hold the leg during passive movement while the other is used to feel for pelvic movement.

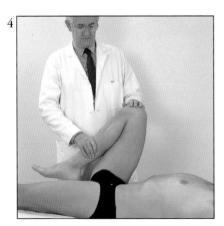

4 Hip flexion is limited by thigh contact with the trunk. It is normally 90 to 100 degrees. It is increased when combined with knee flexion due to relaxation of the hamstring muscles. Forcible passive flexion also increases the range. Some apparent hip flexion is due to flexion of the lumbar spine and pelvic tilting. This can be confirmed by the examiner placing the left hand, palm upwards, behind the lumbar curve during active or passive hip flexion.

5 Abnormalities of the hip joint may limit flexion and the amount of this fixed flexion can be assessed by Thomas' Test for fixed flexion. In this the normal hip is flexed until the lumbar curve is just flattened. This is determined by the left hand placed behind the lumbar spine. At this point, the number of degrees of elevation of the contralateral thigh from the horizontal denotes the degree of fixed flexion.

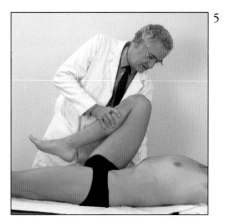

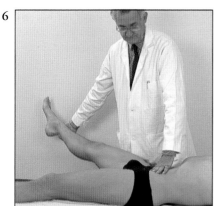

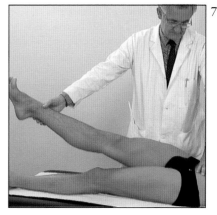

6 and 7 Active and passive abduction and adduction are tested after raising the heel clear of the contralateral leg with the observer's right hand. Pelvic movement is monitored by the observer's left hand, placed on one, or across both anterior superior iliac spines. The movements are respectively, 45 and 30 degrees from a plane at right angles to a line joining the two anterior superior iliac spines.

8 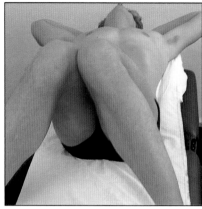 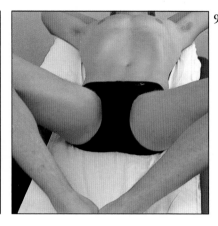 9

8 and 9 Rotation is assessed in flexion and extension. In the former the hip and knee are flexed to 90 degrees and the foot moved medially (external rotation) and laterally (internal rotation). They are respectively 45 and 20 degrees.

10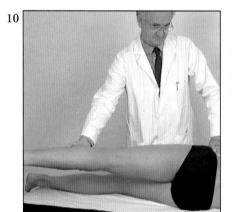

10 Extension of the hip joint is 10 to 20 degrees and can be tested with the patient lying on the contralateral side or lying prone, lifing the bent knee off the couch. Rotation is re-examined in this prone position.

Abnormal mobility of the hip joint may be determined by gripping the flexed thigh with both hands and assessing the presence of any telescopic movement by pulling on the limb.

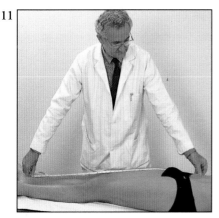
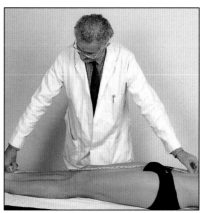

11 and 12   Abnormalities of the hip joint may alter leg length and there may be true or apparent shortening, the latter being due to abnormal tilting of the pelvis. The patient is first asked to lie straight in the bed. True shortening is measured between the anterior superior iliac spine and the medial malleolus on each side or an equivalent position on each knee, such as the medial femoral condyle or patella. Apparent shortening is between the umbilicus or sternal angle and each medial malleolus.

13 Examination is completed by observing the patient standing and walking. The act of standing and stance should be observed for discomfort and disability. When standing on one leg, the opposite side of the pelvis is raised by abduction at the hip joint of the weight-bearing leg. This can be confirmed by an observer standing behind the patient, comparing the buttock creases and palpating the two anterior superior iliac spines. In some hip joint abnormalities, abduction is lost and, on standing on one leg, the opposite side of the pelvis drops, this is know as a positive Trendelenburg test.

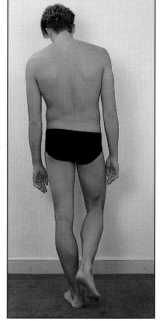

13

Hip joint abnormalities can have marked effect on gait. This can also be produced by musculo-skeletal abnormalities elsewhere in the spine, pelvis and lower limbs, and painful soft tissue conditions. Interpretation is therefore dependent on a detailed general examination, directed by the patient's history.

Note the rhythm and timing of each step, and the pressure applied on each foot. Waddling gaits are produced by inadequate gluteal muscles and congenital dislocation of the hip joint. Other common neurological abnormalities are the shuffling gait of Parkinson's, the spastic hemiplegic, the paralysis of lower motor neurone lesions and incoordination of cerebellar disease.

Knee Joint

Inspection

The neutral position of the knee is in extension and a painful knee is often held in a few degrees of flexion. Compare the two sides. Note skin changes, swelling, deformity, and other changes of contour. Pre- and infrapatellar bursae, popliteal cysts and cartilaginous protrusions along the joint line are common pathologies. Quadriceps wasting is most easily seen by hollows on either side and just above the patella, particularly medially, due to loss of bulk of the lower fibres of the vastus medialis muscle.

Palpation

14

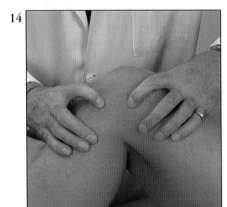

14 Systematically examine the circumference and surface of the patella, the femoral and tibial condyles, and the joint margins. Look for warmth, tenderness and synovial thickening, the latter particularly on either side of the patella, and note any of the lumps mentioned in the previous section. Tears of the medial or lateral ligaments produce tenderness at their proximal and distal attachments, at the femoral and tibial condyles and the upper end of the fibula.

15 Cartilagenous tenderness is along the anterolateral and anteromedial joint line. Crepitus is examined for as considered in movement.

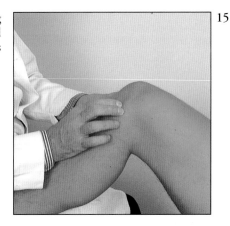

Tests for Effusion

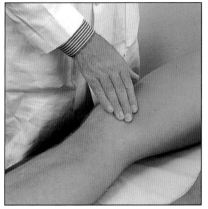

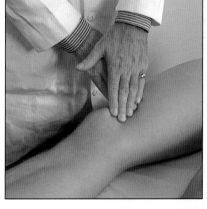

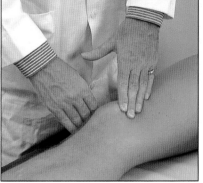

16 to 18 If only a small amount of fluid is present, empty the medial side of the joint by gently sweeping fluid into the suprapatellar pouch. Now sweep down the lateral side of the patella. Small amounts of fluid will pass back into the medial side of the joint, producing a small bulge behind the patella. If the joint is tensely swollen, pressure on one side behind the patella can be felt, transmitted to the other.

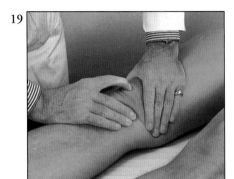

19 The classical test for fluid is the patellar tap. The left hand compresses the lower thigh and slides down towards the patella pushing fluid out of the suprapatellar pouch. This hand is maintained in position above the patella and the right hand used to push the patella back onto the femoral condyles. If fluid is present the patella is separated from the condyles and this pressure produces a bony tap as the patella touches the underlying femur.

Movement

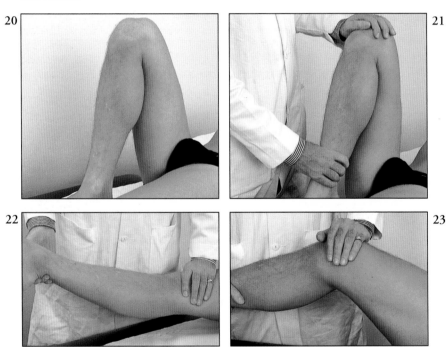

20 to 23 Active flexion is from 0 to 135 degrees, a few more degrees can be obtained by passively compressing calf and thigh muscles. Up to 5 degrees of passive extension may be present. Listen for clicks and creaks. In passive movement, the examiner holds the ankle with the right hand and rests the left hand on the patella to feel for crepitus. This may also be detected by sliding the patella sideways across the femoral condyles.

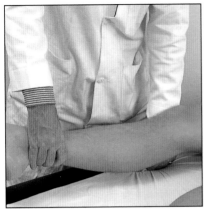 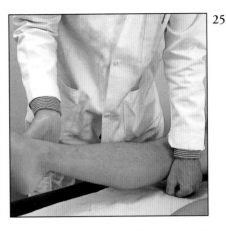

24 and 25 The medial ligament is tested for pain and laxity by placing the left fist on the lateral side of the extended knee. The ankle is gripped with the right hand and an attempt made to abduct the tibia on the femur. The lateral ligament is tested similarly by placing the fist against the medial side of the joint and adduction attempted. In the normal knee neither of these movements should be present.

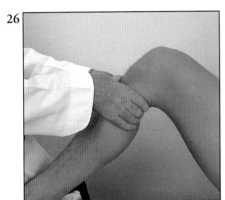 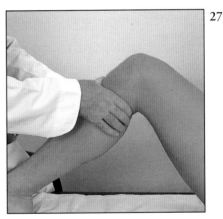

26 and 27 Cruciate ligament function is assessed by the draw test. The knee is flexed to 90 degrees with the foot resting on the couch. The examiner sits on the forefoot and grips the upper end of the calf with both hands and pulls forwards and pushes backwards: there should be no gliding movement. Anterior movement suggests damage of the anterior cruciate ligament and the reverse, the posterior.

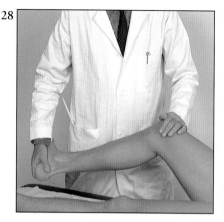 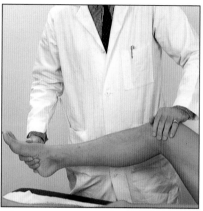

28 and 29 Loose bodies within the knee and damaged menisci may cause locking of the joint. Menisci are assessed in sitting, squatting and standing and by the McMurray test. In the latter, the examiner holds the ankle with the right hand and the knee with the left. The right hand is used to rotate the foot, first in one direction and then in the other. In each case, both hands are used to apply an abduction force across the knee while gradually extending from the flexed position. In the presence of an abnormal cartilage this manoeuvre may produce pain, a click or the protrusion of a lump along the joint margin.

Muscle wasting is assessed by measurement as considered under the general examination of the joints. Examination of the knee is completed by asking the patient to stand up, looking for valgus (knock knees) and varus (bow legs) deformities and observing the gait.

The Ankle and Foot

Inspection

The natural position of the ankle is in slight plantar flexion and slight inversion. The lateral malleolus is a little more prominent and its tip is just distal to that of the medial, the joint line being 1cm above the latter. There may be colour changes, scars, swelling and deformity of all joints. Examine the sole for callosities. A small amount of fluid in the ankle joint presents as puffiness just in front of each malleolus. Larger amounts of fluid fill in the hollow on either side of the tendo Achilles. Other common findings in the foot are: fixed lateral deviation of the main axis of the great toe (hallux valgus), clawing of the toes (fixed flexion deformities) and abnormalities of the transverse and longitudinal arches.

Palpation and Movements

Tenderness and swelling may be localized to the joint or to ligaments or soft tissue abnormality.

30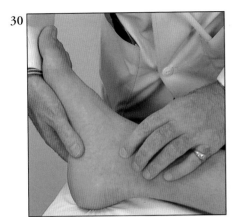

31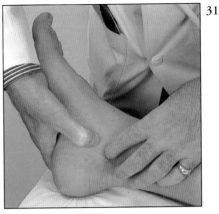

30 and 31 Palpation of the malleoli and the medial and lateral collateral ligaments of the ankle joint is valuable in localising injuries.

32 A transmitted impulse may be obtained between the two sides of the tendo Achilles if sufficient fluid is present.

32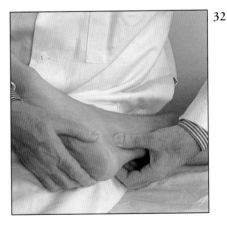

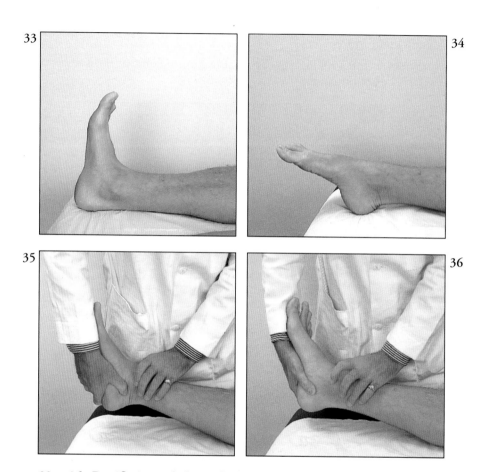

33 to 36 Dorsiflexion and plantar flexion occur primarily at the ankle joint, the former (raising the toes towards the knee) is to 20 degrees and the latter to 50 degrees. Movement of the ankle joint is more lax in plantar flexion when a few degrees of passive abduction and adduction can be obtained. The knee is flexed to reduce calf tension when assessing the degree of fixed flexion deformity of an ankle.

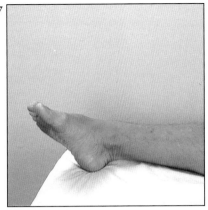
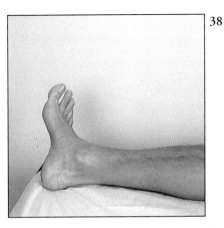

38

37 and 38 Inversion and eversion take place mainly at the subtalar and the talo-calcaneonavicular joints. The calcaneus and the navicular bones carry the fore part of the foot with them.

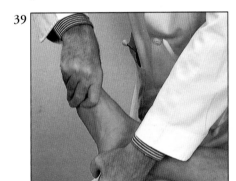
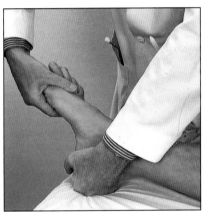

39 and 40 In passive assessment, the observer holds the ankle in the left hand and the forefoot in the right. Inversion, when the sole turns inwards, is to 30 degrees and eversion to 5 degrees.

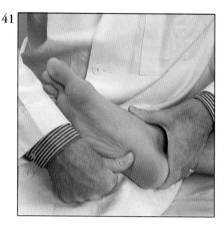 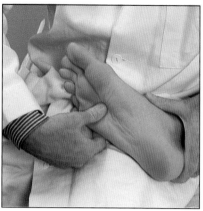

41 and 42 Palpation of the sole may identify deep tenderness. Common conditions are a painful calcaneal spur and injuries of the muscles, bones and ligaments of the sole.

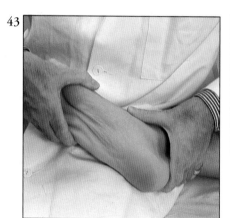 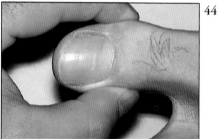

43 and 44 Squeezing across the metatarsophalangeal joints may reveal tenderness, suggestive of inflammatory disorders. Individual interphalangeal joints are assessed by feeling and moving.

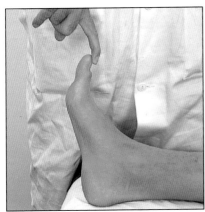

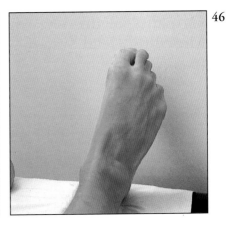

45 and 46 Dorsiflexion and plantar flexion of the metacarpophalangeal joints are respectively 60 and 40 degrees. Flexion of the interphalangeal joints is approximately 60 degrees.

47 A variable small degree of fanning (abduction) of the toes is possible.

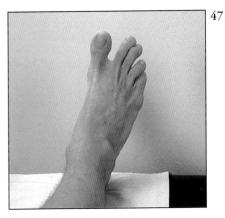

Checklist for the Assessment of the Musculoskeletal System

History

Localise symptomatic bones, joints and muscles

Note: pain, stiffness, limited movement, creaking, cracking, locking, giving way, swelling, wasting, contractures, deformities, loss of function

Manual dexterity: dressing, toiletry, eating, writing

Mobility: ability to sit and stand; walking distance, assistance needed, mechanical aids required; independence

Symptoms of inflammatory disorders: fever, malaise, ocular problems, urethritis, diarrhoea

Examination

General

Cushingoid appearance; pain at rest/on movement; Paget's deformity; weight; fever, malaise, inflammatory eye conditions; blue sclera; gouty tophi; digital trophic changes

Nails: colour, discoloration, pitting, ridging, hyperkeratosis

Local—ensure appropriate exposure

NB compare bones, joints and muscles of the two sides of the body, and record any abnormalities of asymptomatic joints

LOOK:

Skin: creases, scars, colour, erythema, atrophy, rashes, sinuses

Shape: swelling of bone, bursae, synovium, effusions; bony alignment (valgus/varus), subluxation, dislocation; shortening, deformity, wasting

Position: at rest and during activity

Hand deformities: Swan neck; Boutonniere's; Z thumb; finger drop; mallet finger; Dupuytren's contracture; Heberden/Bouchard nodes; ulnar deviation

Posture: kyphoscoliosis; neurological and myopathic abnormalities; Trendelenberg test for congenital hip dislocation

FEEL:

Skin, soft tissue and bones; warmth, tenderness, thickening, nodules, overgrowth, deformity

Abnormal bursae/synovial thickening

Effusions: reducible, fluctuant, ballottable, transillumination

Fractures: tenderness, deformity

Palpate and percuss abnormal nerves

Map out altered cutaneous sensation

MOVE:

Active, passive and resisted movements in each joint plane

Note: pain, power, tone, range, creaking, crepitus, clicking, triggering, locking, hypermobility, telescoping, contractures, stability

Fracture: abnormal mobility, crepitus

Deformity: mobile or fixed

Hand: ability to grip, pinch and do up shirt buttons

Gait: spastic; ataxic; waddling; limp; use of mechanical aids

MEASURE:

Range of joint movements (goniometer)

Limb circumference at equivalent levels from fixed bony points on each side

True and apparent leg shortening, Bryant's triangle

It is usual to proceed to X-ray symptomatic areas in order to identify abnormal bone and soft tissues.

Systemic Investigation

History taking and examination identify the diseased system or systems, and investigation of this system provides supportive evidence of the presence and extent of the abnormality. This section considers the investigations that are helpful in diagnosing abnormalities of each system. Some laboratories may place a different emphasis on the various techniques and new investigations often replace current ones. The section is only intended as a guide to the field.

Investigations may also be used as routine screening tests, taken at such times as examinations for insurance purposes, first attendance at a general practice, hospital out-patients or in-patients, and preoperatively. Examples are urinalysis for the diagnosis of diabetes and renal disease; a full blood count to exclude anaemia and blood dyscrasias; blood urea, electrolytes and glucose; liver function tests, including calcium; an ESR to indicate the presence of systemic disease; and a chest x-ray to diagnose unsuspected chronic pulmonary disorders, especially tuberculosis. Other examples of community screening include mammography and the taking of cervical smears.

In a clinical context, investigations are initiated with a view to answering a specific diagnostic question—either positively making a diagnosis, or excluding it. This is a vital principle to uphold. We are in a defensive era of medical practice, but also an era in which the sequelae of diminishing resources influence our diagnostic approach. Often, the fear of misdiagnosis, and its potential litigious consequences, propel the newly-qualified doctor to request an inappropriate number of investigations—some costly, others potentially dangerous. This approach, while understandable, is to be deplored. At all times, one should be undertaking an investigation specifically to test a particular diagnostic hypothesis. Performing investigations in the absence of such hypotheses often leads to the gathering of irrelevant information and is rarely justified. If in doubt about whether or not to perform a test, the clinician should ask himself or herself whether knowledge of the information obtained will influence patient management.

This chapter covers the more important investigations used in clinical practice. No attempt has been made to be comprehensive—this would be beyond the scope of the book. We have however, attempted to consider diagnostic tests on a systems basis, and at the beginning of each section, we have singled out the key tests pertaining to that section, prior to listing individual investigations.

Investigation of Cardiovascular Disease

The key tests in the initial investigation of suspected cardiovascular disease are the electrocardiogram, the chest x-ray and an echocardiogram. Exercise testing and 24 hour monitoring of cardiac rhythm are also in frequent clinical use. Coronary angiography is reserved for patients with suspected coronary artery disease.

The Electrocardiogram

This simple investigation records the activation and subsequent repolarization of the myocardium. It is an essential part of cardiological workup and is used to identify rhythm disorders and myocardial infarction. Using voltage criteria for the QRS complex, it is possible to determine whether ventricular hypertrophy is present, and ST segment and T wave changes are useful for monitoring electrolyte disturbances, such as hypo- and hyperkalaemia, and hypocalcaemia.

Holter Monitor

Using the Holter monitor (24 hour ECG), the cardiac rhythm can be recorded over a 24–48 hour period onto tape; it is then played back using a decoder. The investigation is particularly useful in the investigation of palpitations, and sudden loss of consciousness. It may reveal both tachycardias and bradycardias, and may be of diagnostic importance.

The Exercise ECG

If myocardial ischaemia (ischaemic heart disease) is suspected, but the base line electrocardiogram is normal, it may be appropriate to stress the patient using a standard exercise protocol during which the electrocardiogram (12 lead) is recorded. As the heart is progressively stressed, with an increase in heart rate and blood pressure, depression of the ST segment may occur which reverses on discontinued exercise. Such ST segment depression has a strong predictive value for underlying significant coronary artery disease.

Echocardiography

Both M mode and two dimensional echocardiograms are now readily available and can be performed at the patient's bedside if necessary. The technique is used to diagnose pericardial fluid, as well as evaluate ventricular function. It is an essential method for picking up abnormalities of the mitral, aortic, pulmonary and tricuspid valves, abnormal thickening of the interventricular septum or left ventricular wall, and diagnosis of congenital heart disease. The Echo Doppler, a modification of the standard echocardiogram, can allow trivial regurgitation and stenosis to be diagnosed where it would not be clinically apparent.

Radioisotope Ventriculography

In this method, a radioactive isotope (usually technetium) is injected into a peripheral vein and a gamma camera, centred over the heart, detects the passage of the radioisotope into the right ventricle, and subsequently into the left ventricle. It is a sensitive method for determining the ejection fraction and investigating contractivity of the heart, as well as the diagnosis of ventricular aneurysms.

Myocardial Scintigraphy

Thallium has similar properties to potassium and is taken up by myocardial cells. In the presence of coronary artery occlusion or obstruction, the area of myocardium served by this coronary vessel will be poorly perfused and, after an intravenous injection of labelled thallium, the isotope picture overlying the ventricular muscle is attenuated. This lack of perfusion may be accentuated during stress, such as exercise, when there is differential blood flow to the unaffected myocardium, showing up as a cold area within the ischaemic tissue.

Cardiac Catheterisation and Angiography

This is an extemely effective way of investigating potential valve failure, measurement of pressures in the atria and ventricles, and is particularly useful for the diagnosis of shunts: in addition, oxygen saturations may be measured. Injection of radio-opaque materials allows the heart chambers to be visualised and this is useful prior to surgical repair.

Coronary Arteriography

This is the investigation of choice in the management of patients with ischaemic heart disease. The severity and probable prognosis of coronary vascular disease is assessed by displaying the extent of the disease and by selective arteriography of the left and right coronary vessels. The femoral artery is usually cannulated, and the catheter tip placed inside the ostia of both the right and left coronary vessel. Left ventricular function is also investigated by separate injection directly into the left ventricular cavity.

Investigation of Respiratory Disease

The key investigations in respiratory medicine are chest x-ray, arterial gases, peak flow rate, and examination of sputum for microbiology and cytology.

Chest Radiography

Chest radiography is the cornerstone of all respiratory investigations. In practice, a PA (postero-anterior) film during full inspiration is performed to detect abnormal lung marking, parenchymal shadowing and masses.

Lung Function Tests

Pulmonary function tests determine:
a) the mechanical characteristics of the ventilatory pump,
b) the adequacy of gas exchange across the alveolar membrane.

A large variety of tests are available but the peak inspiratory flow rate and arterial gas estimation are a useful preliminary means of screening.

Peak Expiratory Flow Rate (PEFR)

This requires the use of a Wright's peak flow meter, and the patient is asked to take a deep inspiration and blow out a maximum expiratory effort through a tube connected to a meter. It is a simple and repro-ducible measurement, and enables a diagnosis of airflow limitation (obstruction) to be made; it is also useful in the management of asthma.

Spirometry

Measurement of FEV_1 (forced expiratory volume) and FVC (full vital capacity).

The volume of air expired during one second in forced expiration can be measured, and compared to the full vital capacity. A normal person will expel over 80% of their full vital capacity within one second. Prolongation of the FEV_1, suggests air flow limitation.

Spirometry also allows the full vital capacity to be measured.

Estimation of Lung Volumes

The volume of gas in the lungs can be calculated by measuring the dilution of a known quantity of an inhaled gas, usually helium. Volumes are reduced in the presence of interstitial disease (restrictive defects) and may be increased where there is air trapping, such as in emphysema.

Diffusion Capacity of the Lung

This measures efficiency of gaseous exchange across the alveolar membrane, and is calculated by monitoring the expiratory and inspiratory concentrations of the inhaled gas (carbon monoxide).

Arterial Gas Estimation

This may be performed by puncturing the radial artery or the brachial artery, usually after infiltration of local anaesthetic. The sample is taken in a small quantity of heparin and, after mixing, stored in ice until the analysis; the sample is then passed into an autoanalyser which measures pO_2, pCO_2 and pH. This is the ultimate test of lung function, and is essential in the evaluation of respiratory insufficiency of any aetiology.

Bronchoscopy

This is the visual examination of the bronchial tree using a flexible fibreoptic instrument. It enables the sub-segmental bronchi to be examined, and is a particularly useful investigation in the diagnosis of bronchial carcinomas, and other causes of haemoptysis.

Transbronchial Lung Biopsy

A biopsy of the interstitium of the lung can be obtained using a narrow wire forceps, guided through the bronchial tree through a bronchoscope. It is particularly useful in the diagnosis of interstitial lung disease, such as fibrosing alveolitis and alveolar cell carcinoma.

Bronchio-Alveolar Lavage

In this investigation, saline is used during bronchoscopy to irrigate particular segments of lung tissue. The lung is then aspirated, and cytological and bacteriological material may be obtained.

Open Lung Biopsy

This is performed through a limited thoracotomy, and is useful in the detailed evaluation of interstitial lung disease.

Transthoracic Lung Biopsy

Biopsy of interthoracic masses may be obtained with a needle, passed through the chest wall under local anaesthetic using x-ray control. It is useful for diagnosis of peripheral carcinomas which may not be accessible to bronchoscopic biopsy.

Pleural Aspiration

This is the procedure whereby pleural fluid is obtained through a needle passed through the chest wall under local anaesthetic. The manoeuvre is particularly useful in the diagnosis of malignancy and infective conditions. It is also therapeutic, as the fluid may be removed from the pleural cavity.

Pleural Biopsy

A biopsy of the parietal pleura can be obtained by passing a special needle (Abrams' needle) through the chest wall under local anaesthetic. It is usually undertaken in a patient with a pleural effusion. The fragments of parietal pleura obtained are useful in the diagnosis of malignancy, mesothelioma, and tuberculosis.

Thoracoscopy

This is direct visualisation of the pleural surfaces with an instrument passed through the chest wall, usually under general anaesthetic. It is usually only performed when there is fluid that separates the pleural surfaces.

Mediastinoscopy

This is the direct visualisation of the mediastinal contents with a rigid instrument passed percutaneously just behind the sternum. It is performed under a general anaesthetic, and may be useful in the diagnosis of mediastinal masses and staging of lung tumours.

Computerised Axial Tomography of the Lungs

Transverse sections of the lungs are compiled using a computer, after imaging at multiple angles using a CT scanner. It is particularly useful in the diagnosis of bronchiectasis, lung cancer, and pulmonary sarcoidosis.

Ventilation Perfusion (VP) Lung Scanning

Isotope scans of the perfusion of a lung can be obtained through intravenous injection of technetium. Isotopic examination of the ventilation pattern can be obtained through the use of an inhaled radiolabelled Krypton. These VQ scans are particularly useful in the diagnosis of pulmonary thromboembolic disease where ventilation patterns may be retained, but there is mismatch with lack of perfusion.

Immunological Tests in Lung Disease

Mantoux/Heaf Test

This comprises the intradermal injection of tuberculin to assess a hypersensitivity response to the microbacterium tuberculosis organism. It is valuable in the diagnosis of previous and active pulmonary, or other forms of tuberculosis.

Kveim Test

This is becoming an obsolete investigation, and comprises the intradermal administration of human sarcoid antigen, the point of biopsy identified by a small ink tatoo which is subsequently biopsied and examined histologically. Cutaneous granuloma formation at the site of intradermal injection suggests active sarcoidosis. Positive tests are usually diagnostic, but the sensitivity is only 25%.

The Intradermal Allergen Test

This constitutes the subcutaneous injection of an allergen such as grass pollen or house dust mite. A positive test produces an immediate weal reaction plus a flare response. It usually signifies the presence of IgE antibodies to the injected antigen.

Radioallergosorbent Test (RAST)

In this investigation, IgE antibody to specific antigens may be identified.

Precipitin Tests

These demonstrate the presence of precipitating antibodies occurring in type 3 immunological responses, typical of extrinsic alveolitidies. This may occur in Farmer's and Bird Fancier's allergic lung.

Bronchial Challenge Tests

These are particularly useful in the diagnosis of occupational asthma caused by various chemicals. Lung function tests are performed, during and after exposure to the suspected inhaled allergen.

Investigation of Gastrointestinal Disease

Radiological investigations of the upper and lower gastrointestinal tract (barium meal and enema) form the backbone of GI investigation. More recently, flexible fibreoptic examination of the upper and lower intestinal tracts has become widespread, and may soon replace totally the more traditional imaging techniques.

Alterations in appetite or bowel habit in the middle and older ages must be considered as the first signs of neoplasia until proved otherwise. Barium studies and/or endoscopy are used to confirm or exclude this or other diagnoses as soon as possible.

The prime clinical abnormality of liver disease is the presence of jaundice with a dark urine, an obstructive pattern and pale stools. Serum bilirubin provides supportive evidence and further serological and haematological tests provide evidence of the type and extent of liver abnormality. Ultrasound is an effective way of diagnosing gallstones and biliary obstruction as well as the presence of hepatic metastases.

Plain Radiography

Abdominal plain radiology, usually with the patient in the erect and supine positions may be useful for the demonstration of dilatated obstructed bowel, with fluid levels. It may also reveal subdiaphragmatic air, suggestive of perforation. It is particulary useful for identification of calcification within the pancreas and in gallstones (about 10%), and gas in the biliary tree.

Barium Swallow

This is an investigation to delineate the oesophagus. Barium sulphate suspension is swallowed and coats the mucosa of the oesophagus. A number of films are taken, and these may show obstruction, ulceration and dilatation of the oesophagus, as well as conditions such as akalasia. Motility problems within the oesophagus can be assessed by this method.

Barium Meal

In this investigation, barium sulphate is swallowed and outlines the stomach. A double contrast film is usually obtained to demonstrate mucosal detail. This requires the swallowing of a tablet which will generate gas within the stomach. The technique is useful in the demonstration of ulcers, tumours, and outlet obstruction to the stomach. Subsequent visualisation of the duodenal cap is useful in the diagnosis of duodenal ulcers or extrinsic compression.

Small Bowel Enema

Barium is introduced through a nasogastric tube directly into the small bowel. This demonstrates the fine mucosal detail of the small intestine, and is useful in the diagnosis of Crohn's disease and other small intestinal conditions.

Barium Enema

In this condition, following a thorough evacuation of the bowel and colonic washout, barium solution and air are introduced into the rectum and colon; this may enable the demonstration of tumours, inflammatory bowel disease, such as Crohn's and ulcerative colitis, and diverticular disease.

Gastrointestinal Endoscopy

Upper GI Endoscopy

This is performed through a flexible endoscope swallowed by the patient, usually after local anaesthetic has been applied to the back of the throat. Patients may require sedation during the procedure. It allows visualisation of the oesophagus and stomach. The instrument may then be passed through the pyloric canal and into the duodenum to inspect the first and second parts for ulceration. The technique enables biopsy of any lesions in the upper gut.

Colonoscopic Examination

An endoscope is passed after the patient has had complete evacuation of the bowel and a colonic washout. The instrument can be passed as far as the terminal ileum, and enables total visualization of the mucosa with biopsy and, where appropriate, therapeutic procedures such as endoscopic polypectomy. Biopsies of the terminal few centimetres of the small intestine may also be performed.

ERCP—Endoscopic Retrograde Cholangio-Pancreatography

This method allows radiographic studies of the pancreatic and biliary ducts. A side-viewing endoscope is passed into the duodenum, the Ampulla of Vater identified, and a catheter introduced into it to cannulate the pancreatic and biliary ducts. Contrast material may then be injected into either or both of these ducts. Stones may be removed through this procedure and sphincterotomy undertaken.

Sigmoidoscopy

This may be performed with either a rigid or flexible instrument, allowing inspection of the rectum and sigmoid colon. It is particularly useful for biopsy of the mucosa, and in the diagnosis of rectal and sigmoid tumours. It can be performed easily as an out-patient procedure without requiring a bowel preparation.

Small Bowel/Jejunal Biopsy

This is performed in the diagnosis of malabsorption or parasitic infestation of the upper gut. A Crosby capsule can be introduced and swallowed. Suction on the tube attached to the capsule releases a small blade, which amputates a fragment of mucosa. The mucosa is then examined under a low power microscope, fixed, sectioned and stained. Biopsies can also be performed using a flexible endoscopic apparatus, although the biopsies are much smaller.

Gastric function test

This is usually performed first thing in the morning in the fasting state. The stomach is intubated with a nasogastric tube and gastric juice collected over 15 minute intervals. A basal output is obtained, and Pentagastrin (6mcg/kg) is then given intramuscularly to stimulate further secretion (to generate maximum acid output). In the Zollinger-Ellison syndrome, basal secretory rates are elevated but not increased after Pentagastin administration.

Tests of Small Bowel Function

Faecal Fat Excretion

Faecal fatty acid excretion may be determined from a timed collection of faeces over a two to three day period following a fixed oral intake of fat. Normal faecal fat excretion is usually <18 mmol/24h and, when this is exceeded, steatorrhea occurs.

Xylose Excretory Test

An oral dose of xylose (5mg) is given, and the urinary excretion of this compound determined. If urine levels are low, this suggests malabsorption, although this can be confounded by the effects of age and deteriorating renal function. Usually, within 2 hours of oral administration, more than 23% of the dose is excreted and more than 35% after 5 hours.

Lactose Tolerance Test

This is used to determine the presence of primary or secondary lactose deficiency. Lactose (50g) is administered orally, and the subsequent rise in blood glucose level is measured. This normally exceeds 1.1 mmols/litre.

Radioisotope and Hydrogen Breath Tests

This is of particular value in the diagnosis of small bowel bacterial contamination (e.g. stagnant loop syndrome and diverticulae). 14C glycocolate is given orally, and any subsequent release of 14C carbon dioxide measured in the breath. When this breath release is premature, it suggests bacterial breakdown of the labelled glycine conjugate in the upper gut. This contrasts with the normal (later) breakdown of conjugate due to entry of the compound into the large intestine.

Hydrogen Breath Test

Following an oral dose of non-absorbable carbohydrate (lactulose) the timing of the peak concentration of hydrogen in the breath is measured. Early increase in hydrogen secretion suggests small bowel overgrowth with bacteria.

Liver Function Tests

Synthetic Liver Function Test

This is performed by measuring the prothrombin time and the albumin level. Many clotting factors (2, 7, 9, 10) are synthesised within the liver, and hepato-cellular dysfunction may lead to inadequate synthesis of these factors, with prolongation of the clotting times.

Serum bilirubin is raised in haemolytic, hepatic and obstructive jaundice, while serum alkaline phosphatase will also be raised in hepatocellular and obstructive liver disease. Serum globulins are raised in chronic liver disease of many causes. A rise in aspartate amino-transaferase (AsT) and alanine amino-transferase (AlT) levels usually signifies hepatocellular dysfunction. Gamma-glutamyl transpeptidase is elevated in hepatocellular disease and obstruction, and easily induced and raised in chronic alcoholism.

Serological Tests in Liver Disease

Alpha Fetoprotein

This is raised in over half the number of patients with hepatoma: however, there may be mild elevations with nodular regeneration in cirrhotic liver disease.

Anti-Nuclear Factor

This may be raised in chronic active hepatitis, as may be smooth muscle antibody. Antimitrochondral (M2, M4) antibody is usually raised in primary biliary cirrhosis.

Serological Markers

The presence of hepatocellular dysfunction, in association with persistent hepatitis surface and core antigens (HB_sA_g, HB_eA_g), and signifies underlying hepatitis B mediated chronic active hepatitis. A number of tests are now available for antibodies to hepatitis C, which may also induce chronic liver disease and predispose to hepatoma.

Ultrasonic Scan of the Liver

This is a simple, cheap and extremely effective investigation. For the jaundiced patient, it will distinguish between parenchymal liver disease and that due to extrahepatic biliary tract obstruction. The technique is also useful in the diagnosis of liver metastases, hepatic abscesses and cysts, and will show up cirrhosis of the liver as well as gallstones.

Liver Biopsy

This is required in the investigation of parenchymal hepatic disease or in hepatic enlargement of uncertain cause. Biopsy is performed under local anaesthesia through a right intercostal space. Either a Menghini or a Trucut needle can be used. The patient clotting status must be satisfactory and platelet count must be normal prior to performing such a procedure.

Tests for Pancreatic Function
Lundh Test Meal

Following a liquid artificial meal, the secretion of pancreatic trypsin, amylase and bicarbonate can be measured after duodenal intubation. Alternatively, a duodenal aspirate can be collected following pancreatic stimulation with intravenous secretin/pancreazymin. However, in this test, gastric secretions must be removed by continuous gastric suction through a nasogastric tube. In chronic pancreatic disease, reduced levels of enzymes and bicarbonate will be found in the pancreatic juice.

Tubeless Test for Pancreatic Function

These depend on the measurement of substances found in the urine which are released by pancreatic enzymes from their parent compounds, e.g. amino-benzoic acid test (trypsin activity) and fluorescein dilaurate (test of lipase activity), as part of the pancreo-laurate test. Ultrasonic and computerised axial tomography of the pancreas are useful for the detection of tumours and pseudocysts. A plain x-ray of the abdomen may show pancreatic calcificiation.

Visceral Angiography

The various arterial trunks supplying the gut (coeliac, superior and inferior mesenteric) may be cannulated and selectively perfused with contrast medium. These are useful investigations for determining the site of alimentary bleeding. The technique is also valuable in the investigation of patients with refractory hypertension, to diagnose renal artery stenosis and adrenal tumours.

Investigation of Genitourinary Disease

Urine analysis for protein and glucose, urine microscopy, culture and sensitivity and urea, creatinine and electrolytes are fundamental investigations of the genitourinary system.

The plasma urea and creatinine are the most commonly used tests of renal function: they are raised in renal failure. The mid-stream urine examination (MSU) is used to look for urinary tract infection. A suprapubic aspirate may be required in a child, since there is danger of contaminants being present through incorrect collection techniques. The glomerular filtration rate can be calculated from timed 24 hour urine collection for urine creatinine and simultaneous serum creatinine level.

$$\text{Creatinine clearance (in ml/min)} = \frac{UV}{P}$$

where U is the urine creatinine, V the urine volume and P the plasma creatinine.

EDTA Clearance

Some radiopharmaceuticals are excreted by the kidney: this may be by glomerular filtration, tubular excretion or the combination of both. A chromium labelled chelate of ethylene diamine tetra-acetic acid ([51Cr]-EDTA) is commonly used to measure the glomerular filtration rate. Blood samples are taken to measure the rate of clearance of the radiopharmaceutical. These products may also provide an image of the kidney using a gamma camera, for example [99mTc]-DTPA scan. In the case of renal artery stenosis, the reduced perfusion of the affected kidney can be accentuated by the administration of 25 mg of Captopril.

Although the current emphasis in urological investigation is towards imaging techniques (ultrasound, radionucleid, CT, MRI, angiography), the IVU and visualisation of the bladder by cystoscopy are still widely available and form important baseline investigations.

Other investigations include seminal analysis in infertility, urodynamic investigations of the lower urinary tract and intracavernosal injection of papaverine in the assessment of impotence.

Investigation of Endocrine Disease

Endocrine Pancreas

A random blood glucose exceeding 11mmol/l is diagnostic of diabetes mellitus. Hypoglycaemia, when associated with symptoms of neuroglycopenia, is usually associated with a blood sugar of less than 2.2mmol/l.

Oral Glucose Tolerance Tests

Following an overnight fast, 75g of glucose are given orally. Blood tests for sugar levels are taken at half hourly intervals for 2 hours. Impaired glucose tolerance is present when the 2 hour post-glucose load is between 7 and 11 mmol/l, whereas a level exceeding 11 mmol/l is pathognomonic of established diabetes mellitus.

Insulin and C Peptide Levels

These are useful in the diagnosis of spontaneous hypoglycaemia, when a low blood sugar will be accompanied by elevated (inappropriate) levels of insulin and C peptide.

Glycosylated Haemoglobin and Fructosamine

Glucose in the blood reacts with haemoglobin and this glycosylated haemoglobin (HbA1c) can be used to estimate the diabetic control over the previous two to three months. In haemolytic disease levels are abnormally low, because red cell turnover is increased. Similarly the test may be unreliable in chronic renal disease. Fructosamine represents a glycosylated albumin and, since the latter is turned over rapidly (weeks), it may be a useful test of glycaemic control over the short term (2 to 3 weeks).

Investigation of Thyroid Disease

A baseline estimation in blood of thyroid stimulating hormone (TSH) and free thyroxine and tri-iodothyronine (FT4 and FT3), is usually adequate to establish whether there is hyper- or hypo-functioning of the thyroid. When FT4 and FT3 are at the upper limit of normal, and the TSH is not fully suppressed, it may be appropriate to perform a thyroid releasing hormone (TRH) test (200 mcg IV). In thyrotoxicosis, there is usually a flat TSH response to this provocative test.

Radioisotope Scans

Technetium pertetnetate may be administered intravenously in patients with goitres. In Grave's disease (diffuse goitre) there is uniformly increased uptake of the radionuclide, which mimics iodine, in that it is trapped by a membrane. Cold nodules have a 10% chance of being malignant. Hot nodules may represent a toxic adenoma, and usually in this instance, the remainder of the thryoid is cold, because TSH has been switched off by negative feedback.

Ultrasound Scanning of the Thyroid

This is useful to distinguish between solid and cystic masses within the thyroid.

Serological Tests for Thyroid Antibodies

The presence of antibodies to thyrogloblin and the microsomal antigen (thyroid peroxidase) is classical of autoimmune thyroid disease. The thyroid simulating antibodies are less frequently sought clinically.

Tests of Adrenal Medullary Function

These are used in the suspected diagnosis of tumour secretion of the catecholamines noradrenaline, adrenaline and dopamine. The simplest test consists of a timed 24 hour urinary collection in 6N HCl for the estimation of urinary free catecholamines. Plasma catecholamines are usually raised in phaeochromocytomas, but their measurement presents several technical difficulties.

Tests of Adrenocortical Function

Tests for Addison's Disease

In primary adrenal insufficiency (Addison's disease), the adrenocorticotrophic hormone (ACTH) is elevated and cortisol fails to rise following the provocative stimulus of giving Tetracosactrin (250mcg IM). In Addison's disease due to autoimmune disease, there may be antibodies to adrenal cortical cells.

Diagnosis of Cushing's Syndrome

Urinary free cortisols are invariably raised in Cushing's syndrome. The oral administration of dexamethazone (low and high dose) may distinguish between pituitary dependent Cushing's disease, and Cushing's syndrome due to either ectopic ACTH or adrenal adenomas/carcinomas.

The corticotrophin releasing factor (CCRF) test given intravenously (100mcg) usually leads to an exaggerated ACTH and cortisol response in cases of Cushing's disease, whereas in adrenal ademonas and ectopic ACTH secretion, the cortical response is usually flattened.

Pituitary Function Tests

The insulin tolerance test (IV 0.15 units/kg) is a dynamic test of cortisol and growth hormone reserve. In order for the test to be valid, the blood glucose must fall to less than 2.2 mmol/l, and the patient must experience symptomatic hypoglycaemia.

Tests for Acromegaly

The classical test is an oral glucose tolerance test, which in normal individuals should lead to complete suppression of growth hormone. In 50% of patients with acromegaly there is a paradoxical rise in growth hormone or simply non-suppression of growth hormone levels.

Tests of Hypothalamo-Pituitary/Gonadal Axis

The simplest test is the measurement of leuteinising/follicular stimulating hormones (LH/FSH) together with either Oestradiol, or Testosterone. In primary gonadal failure, the LH/FSH will be raised and the sex steroid reduced.

In females, a day 21 progesterone will disclose whether a luteal phase is present.

Tests for Metabolic Bone Disease

The usual analyses are: unoccluded serum calcium, plasma phosphate, alkaline phosphatase and parathormone (PTH) estminations.

In primary hyperparathyroidism there is hypercalcaemia and the PTH is usually raised, whereas in other causes of hypercalcaemia, PTH may be suppressed by the elevated calcium.

25-hydroxy vitamin D3 and 1,25-dihydroxycholecalciferol are reduced in malabsorption and in later cases of renal failure. Urinary calcium excretion is normally less than 6 mmols per 24 hours, it may be raised in primary hyperparathyroidism and lowered in cases of malabsorption.

Bone Biopsy

This is usually performed by removing a core of bone from the iliac crest under local anaesthetic. It is a useful way of establishing the diagnosis of oesteomalacia.

Investigation of Rheumatological Disease

Measurement of uric acid, the ESR and serological tests for rheumatoid factor and anti DNA antibodies are the key investigations in rheumatological practice. Radiological assessment of joints plays an important role in defining the specific arthropathy.

Serological Tests

The rheumatoid factor may be measured, as can antinuculear antibodies, double DNA antibodies, and various antibodies to extractable nuclear antigens.

Excess synovial fluid may be aspirated and analysed under the microscope for investivation of possible crystal synovitis.

Arthroscopy may be performed to inspect the joint interior, the knee being the most commonly investigated joint. Serum uric acid is usually raised in gouty conditions.

Investigation of Neurological Disease

The introduction of computerised tomography (CT scan) has revolutionised the investigation of the central nervous system, markedly reducing the need for lumbar punctures and carotid angiography, and making ventriculography obsolete. Magnetic resonance imaging (MRI), isotope scanning and transcranial doppler have further increased the means of non-invasive assessment. The symptoms of cerebrovascular disease are often produced by stenosis across the common carotid bifurcation and cervical ultrasound is a simple and reliable means of screening these vessels.

Lumbar Puncture

This is performed with the patient lying horizontally on the left side, with a flexed neck, trunk and knees. After infiltration with local anaesthetic, a needle is inserted into the lumbar subarachnoid space usually between the L4 and L5 spines. The cerebrospinal fluid (CSF) should begin clear, and the pressure is normally between 50 and 200 mm of fluid. CSF is usually examined for cells, glucose, protein and immunoglobulin content, as well as serology.

CT/MRI Scanning

Structure of the brain can be easily imaged by these techniques. Although the latter is more expensive, it gives better resolution of intracranial structures: it is particularly useful in the diagnosis of tumours and demyelination.

Electroencephalograpy (EEG)

Using a series of electrodes placed on the scalp, the electrical activity of the underlying brain may be recorded. Various normal rhythms can be documented (alpha, theta) depending on their frequency (alpha 8–13, theta 4–7 cycles per second). The technique is useful in the diagnosis of epilepsy and of other localised pathologies.

Sensory Evoked Potentials

The visually evoked response tests the integrity of the optic pathways from the retina, through the optic chiasm and optic tracts, to the lateral geniculate bodies and to the visual cortex. Delay in conduction may occur in patients with multiple sclerosis, pituitary tumours and unsuspected optic neuritis. In auditory evoked responses, following an auditory stimulus, the potentials may be recorded over the auditory cortex.

In somatosensory evoked potentials, following a peripheral stimulus, conduction over the spinal cord may be evaluated as well as the somatosensory cortex.

Electromyography

This is performed by inserting a fine needle into the muscle. The amplified potential difference can be displayed on an oscilloscope. Healthy muscle is electrically silent, but if denervation has occured, low amplitude, short duration potentials may be elicited, accompanied clinically by fasciculation. In muscle disease, on muscle contraction, there may be general reduction in action potentials with broken short duration complexes. In denervated muscle, single high amplitude potentials are registered.

Conduction Velocities

The speed of electrical conduction along a nerve can be measured by applying an electrical stimulus at one end, and measuring the time taken to produce an evoked potential. Reduction of nerve conduction velocity occurs in the presence of nerve compression or demyelination processes. Both motor and sensory potentials can be measured using skin electrodes. In the adult, the normal velocity is 50–60 metres per second in the median, ulnar and radial nerves. This can be markedly reduced in the presence of demyelination. In the presence of axonal degeneration, surviving axons conduct at normal rate but the evoked muscle potentials are reduced.

Radioisotope Brain Scan

The distribution of radioactivity over the scalp may be recorded following an intravenous injection of technetium 99mTc. Increased vascularity of areas of the brain where there is a break in the blood/brain barrier may show increased uptake. This may occur in secondary deposits and some infarcts.

Myelography

In this procedure, contrast medium is injected into the subarachnoid space following a lumbar puncture. The contrast medium can be made to move along the spinal canal by suitably altering the patient's position. An x-ray is taken to demonstrate potential compression on the cord anywhere from the base of the skull to the sacral area.

Muscle Biopsy

Under local anaesthetic, a piece of muscle, usually from the deltoid or quadriceps (vastus lateralis), can be taken for histological and histochemical examination. In the case of muscle disease, the biopsy should be taken from an involved but not wasted muscle. Changes may be those of denervation, with patchy wasting of fibres, or myositis, where there is an increased inflammatory cell number, together with muscle fibre damage.

Peripheral Nerve Biopsy

This may be used in the investigation of a peripheral neuritis. The sural nerve is the preferred site and can be biopsied by administering local anaesthetic behind the lateral malleolus and then dissecting down to the nerve. A small fragment is removed for histological and histochemical analysis.

Cerebral Angiography

Contrast medium is introduced through a direct carotid puncture or via a catheter introduced through the femoral artery. In the latter, images can be obtained of the aortic arch, or selectively, of the carotid, subclavian and vertebral arteries. X-rays are taken during the arterial phase and subsequent venous phases of the cerebral circulation. The investigation is particularly useful for detecting aneurysms, and abnormal circulation due to angiomas or tumours.

Digital Subtraction Angiography

This technique gives a similar picture to conventional cerebral arteriography but uses an intravenous bolus injection or a reduced volume of intra-arterial contrast medium.

MRI Angiography

Cerebral vessels may be demonstrated by IV injection of contrast medium during MRI scanning. The advantages of a non-invasive technique are dependent on the subject remaining very still, during what can be a long examination period.

Investigation of Haematological Disorders

A full blood count, serum iron and total iron binding capacity (TIBC), B_{12} and folate are the basic tests.

Full Blood Count

This is normally an automated estimation of haemoglobin, red cell indices, white cell count, the differential count and the platelet count. Modern counters can also give information on the size and form of red cells and platelets. Absolute values and red cell indices include the red cell count, the packed cell count (haematocrit), the mean cell haemoglobin and the mean cell volume.

Examination of the Blood Film

This is an essential investigation for the diagnosis of many blood disorders, and enables an analysis of the morphology of red and white cells, and platelets. Anisocytosis is the name given to differences in the size of red cells; poikilocytosis designates the difference in shape of the cells; microcytosis designates small red cells, characteristic of thalassemias, some other haemoglobinopathies, and classical iron deficiency anaemia; macrocytosis designates large red cells, classically found in megaloblastic anaemias, refractory anaemias, myelodysplasia, liver disease and hypothyroidism.

Reticulocytes are large red cells. Hypochromia is the term used to describe reduced haemoglobin concentration and is usually found in association with microcytosis. Spherocytosis designates small, dark, round cells, which lack the characteristic biconcavity of red cells. It may be found in congenital spherocytosis and other autoimmune anaemias. Schistocytosis is the term given to the presence of fragmented red cells, usually found in haemolytic anaemias particularly microangiopathic processes.

Target cells are found in some haemoglobinopathies, liver disease, iron deficiency anaemia and following splenectomy. Acanthocytosis describes the presence of crenated red cells, found in some congenital abnormalities. Polychromasia is the bluish staining of some red cells, usually associated with an increased reticulocyte count. Howell-Jolly bodies designate the dark staining dots found in red cells, which represent nuclear remnants. They may be found in a number of dyserythropoietic anaemias.

Estimation of Blood Volume

In this situation, it is usual to use an isotope dilution technique with red cells being labelled with Chromium ^{51}Cr and plasma with ^{125}I labelled albumin. The technique is useful in the diagnosis of polycythaemia.

Bone Marrow Aspirate/Trephine

This is an important investigation in the diagnosis of several blood disorders, particularly neoplasia. Aspiration of the blood marrow is performed to assess red cell and white cell morphology; the preferred site being the sternum. A trephine biopsy is useful to assess the cellularity in marrow histology, and is essential in the investigation of aplastic anaemia or malignant infiltration of the bone marrow. The most commonly used site is the posterior iliac crest. The marrow aspirate can be cultured, particularly if chronic infection with tuberculosis or brucellosis is suspected.

Carboxy-Haemoglobin

This is normally present in only trace amounts in normal individuals, but may be increased by more than 15% in smokers. It may be useful in the diagnosis of mild polycythaemia.

Cell Marker Studies

These are particularly useful in the identification of malignant white cells, and enable the classification of disease, particularly leukaemias and lymphomas. Cell markers are antigens present on the surface of the cells which are usually typed by the use of monoclonal antibodies. Some antigens may only be present on premature cells and disappear as the cells mature. There is a specific set of lymphoid cell markers. For example, in acute lymphoblastic leukaemia of childhood the CALL antigen may be present, this being an early lymphoid marker. The surface membrane immunoglobulin (SmIG) is a B cell marker. Some markers are particularly useful in monitoring the progress of acquired immunodeficiency (AIDS) disease, where the determination of T4/T8 cell counts have important prognostic significance.

Chromosome Analysis (Karyography)

This is useful in the diagnosis of genetic disease such as Down's syndrome, Klinefelter's syndrome and certain haematological diseases, particularly chronic myelocytic leukaemia, where the Philadelphia chromosome may be found. In the investigation of translocations, high resolution G (Giemsa) banding is necessary for precise localisation.

Cytochemistry

This has been used for the identification of leukaemic blast cells. The stains usually identify intracellular enzymes or other cytoplasmic components.

Acid Phosphate

This picks up particularly T cells. Esterase is useful in distinguishing between myeloblasts and monocytoblasts. Myeloperoxidase is useful for characterising myeloblasts.

Neutrophil Alkaline Phosphatase

This is characteristically low or absent in chronic granulocytic leukaemia but raised in leukaemoid reactions (i.e. shift to the left in acute infective episodes). Periodic acid-Schiff (PAS) stains intracellular glycogen and gives a black positivity, characteristically seen in lymphoblasts. Sudan black is useful in the investigation of potential myeloblastic leukaemias. Terminal transferase (TdT) is present in undifferentiated lymphoblasts. It is particularly useful in the differentiation of lymphoblastic and myeloblastic leukaemia.

2,3-DPG (Diphosphoglycerate)

This important red cell metabolite determines the position of the oxygen dissociation curve. Its depletion causes the oxygen dissociation curve to move to the left, whereas an increase moves it to the right. The test is used in the diagnosis of certain rare types of polycythaemia, haemoglobinopathies and red cell enzyme defects.

Typical Normal Values

Specimens must be collected under the appropriate condition, for example with the subject fasting or from a non-occluded arm. When in doubt discuss these matters with the laboratory, particularly for non-routine investigations.

Follow the hospital protocol for the size of sample and the recommended container. Dispose of the syringe and needle in the containers provided, making sure they are not a hazard to yourself or any other worker.

The specimen must be fully labelled, this includes the hospital number as well as the patient's name, thus avoiding any confusion between patients with the same name. A request form should be similarly fully labelled and all requested information provided. It is the responsibility of the individual collecting the specimen to make sure that it reaches the laboratory. Whatever the prescribed routine, ensure that during this transfer specimens are appropriately stored and are not a hazard to anyone in transit.

If a test needs doing the result is worthy of following up. Read typed reports or information on a VDU carefully, as mistakes can have lethal effects. In an emergency, results may be obtained by telephone but check the subsequent hard copy. All reports should be initialled by the doctor concerned before filing in the patient's notes.

Laboratories can vary in their published normal values. The following list provides typical norms but local standards should be used when interpreting hospital reports.

Tests: Blood

Acid Phosphatase	<5.0 iu/l
ACTH	<10–80 ng/l
Albumin	35–50 g/l
Aldosterone	Recumbent:
	100–550 pmol/l
	Ambulant:
	900–1500 pmol/l
Alkaline Phosphatase	35 –130 iu/l
Amylase	<300 iu/l
Antidiuretic Hormone	2 –6 pmol/l

Apo Lipoprotein A1	0.7–1.7 mg/l
Apo Lipoprotein A2	0.2–0.6 mg/l
Apo Lipoprotein B	0.6–1.4 mg/l
Bicarbonate	24–30 mmol/l
Bilirubin	3–17 μmol/l
Calcitonin	<0.08 μgl
Calcium (corrected)	2.20–2.65 mmol/l
Chloride	95–105 mmol/l
Cholesterol	Age and sex related
	Adults in range:
	3.0–5.6 mmol/l
Cortisol	at 09:00: 200–650 nmol/l
	at 24:00: 30-120 nmol/l
Creatinine	60–120μmol/l
Dihydrotestosterone	in Adult Males:
	1.0–2.9 nmol/l
FSH	Males: 0.5–6.0 lU/l
	Females, Cyclical:
	- early: 2–8 U/l
	- mid: 6–25 U/l
	- luteal: 2–6 U/l
	- menop: 10–50 U/l
Gases (Arterial)	
pH	7.38–7.42
pCO_2	4.5–6.0 kPa
pO_2	11–15 kPa
Gastrin	<40 pmol/l
Glucagon	<50 pmol/l
Glucose (fasting)	3.5–5.5 mmol/l
Growth Hormone (fasting)	<10 mU/l
HBD	40–140 iu/l
HDL Cholesterol	Males: 0.9–1.7 mmol/l
	Females: 1.0–2.2 mmol/l
Ig[F1]	Males: 9–46 nmol/l
	Females: 12 - 48 nmol/l
Iron	13–31 μmol/l
Iron Binding Capacity (total)	40–80 μmol/l
Lipoprotein lipase	5–25 mmol/h
Lithium (therapeutic)	0.7–1.4 mmol/l

Magnesium	0.7–1.0 mmol/l
Neurotensin	<100 pmol/l
Oestradiol	Prepuber.: 37–92 pmol/l
	Males: 55–92 pmol/l
	Females Cyclical:
	- early: 110–183 pmol/l
	- mid: 550–1650 pmol/l
	- luteal: 550–845 pmol/l
	- menop: <200 pmol/l
Osmolality	275–300 mmol/kg
Pancreatic Polypeptide	<300 pmol/l
Phosphate	0.75–1.50 mmol/l
Potassium	3.5–5.0 mmol/l
Progesterone	Males: aver. 2.0 nmol/l
	Females, Cyclical:
	- early: <5 nmol/l
	- luteal: 20–80 nmol/l
17OH-Progesterone	Prepubertal: <1.1 nmol/l
	Males: 0.6–6.0 nmol/l
	Females, Cyclical:
	- early: 0.6–3.0 nmol/l
	- luteal: 3–12 nmol/l
Prolactin	30–400 mU/l
Protein	60–80 g/l
PTH	10–55 pg/ml
Reverse T3	250–650 pmol/l
Salicylate (therapeutic)	<200 mg/l
SGOT	20–40 iu/l
SHBG	Males: 10–50 nmol/l
	Females: 30–90 nmol/l
Sodium	135–45 mmol/l
Somatostatin	<120 pmol/l
TBG	7–17 g/l
Testosterone	Males: 9–30 nmol/l
	Females: 0.5–2.5 nmol/l
Thyroxine (total)	70–140 nmol/l
Triglycerides	Males: 0.7–2.2 mmol/l
	Females: 0.6–1.7 mmol/l
Tri-iodothyronine	1.2–3.0 nmol/l

TSH	0.5–4.7 mU/l
Urea	2.5–6.7 mmol/l
Uric Acid	0.12–0.42 mmol/l
VIP	<30 pmol/l
25OH Vitamin D	19–107 nmol/l
Xylose (25g XTT)	2.0–4.0 mmol/l

Tests: Urine

ADH	10–20 pmol/l
Aldosterone	10–50 nmol/24h
Calcium	2.5–7.5 mmol/24h
Cortisol	Males: <350 nmol/l
	Females: <290 nmol/l
Creatinine	9–18 mmol/24h
HIAA	5–75 μmol/24h
HMMA (VMA)	10–35 μmol/24h
Magnesium	3–5 mmol/24h
Nor-Adrenaline	0.53–1.80 μmol/24hr
Osmolality	40–1400 mosm/kg
Oxalate	30–240 μmol/24h
17 Oxosteroids	20–65 μmol/24h
pH	4.5–7.8
Phosphate	15–50 mmol/24h
Potassium	40–120 mmol/24h
Protein	<0.05 g/l
Sodium	100–250 mmol/24h
Urea	170–600 mmol/24h
Uric Acid	3.0–12.0 mmol/24h
Xylose (25g XTT)	30–50 mmol/5h

Tests: CSF

Glucose	2.8–4.5 mmol/l
Protein	0.1–0.4 g/l

Tests: Faecal Fat

Faecal fat	<18 mmol/24h

Haematology

		Male	Female
Hb	(g/dl)	14.0–17.7	12.2–15.2
PCV	(l/l)	0.42–0.53	0.36–0.45
RBC	(x10^{12}/l)	4.5–6.0	3.9–5.1

MCV	(fl)	80–96
RDW	(%)	less than 14
MCH	(pg)	27–33
MCHC	(g/dl)	32–35
WBC	(x10^9/l)	4.0–11.0
PLATS	(x10^9/l)	150–400
PCT	(%)	0.160–0.350
MPV	(fl)	6.7–10.4
PDW	(%)	less than 17.5

The Patient Record

Accurate note keeping is an essential part of clinical management. It provides a record of what has been found and the action taken. This can subsequently be referred to by the clinician or a colleague, ensuring coordinated continuity of care. Records should be made at the time of history taking and examination, as details are soon forgotten and easily misquoted. Documentation takes time, but it does provide a moment for reflection, often allowing clarification of thoughts and ideas.

The notes should be complete and comprehensive, yet easily read and as concise as possible. They must make sense not only to the recorder but also to other health care workers. This requires a good deal of organisation and discipline, following a set format. These documents have medico-legal significance and therefore must be legible: avoid comments of a personal nature such as those indicating hostility towards, or passing moral judgment on, a patient.

Many specialist units will have a printed history and examination form to be filled in. If this is not available, follow the headings already advised. Start by checking that the notes belong to the patient concerned. If they are blank, record the patient's name, date of birth, address, occupation, and marital status. Note the date of the assessment and the history under the usual six headings, indenting and underlining as appropriate. Begin with the present complaint and past history; followed by drugs and allergies, and social history; finally the family history and systemic review.

Under the examination record the general appearance—whether the patient is anaemic, dyspnoeic, cyanosed, jaundiced, has any significant lymphadenopathy or generalised oedema; record pulse and blood pressure. There follows examination of the system of interest and a systemic review. Record the blood pressure and other measurements such as urinanalysis at the time of these examinations, to ensure accurate reporting. Measurements should be in centimetres rather than related to one's favourite fruits. Although helpful, the latter are imprecise measures. Diagrams, possibly on a regional anatomical stamp, are helpful.

Simple diagrams should be used to record clinical findings, measurements being added when appropriate. When a clinician routinely deals with one area of the body, it is convenient to have a dedicated stamp, onto which can be added clinical findings. Page 256 includes some typical examples: they may be reproduced if required.

The vocal cords are observed by direct or indirect laryngoscopy. The double circles denote proctological findings, the outer is the anal margin

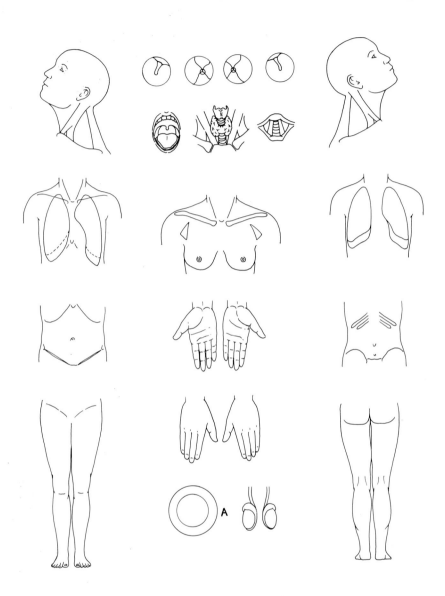

and the inner the muco-cutaneous junction—the 'A' indicates the anterior position; it would be at 12 o'clock if the examination had been undertaken in the lithotomy position.

The anterior and posterior dermatomes (p 160) are often needed in neurological practice and the body for dermatological records. In rheumatology, an homunculus of the whole body, or regions of the body, with circles denoting the joints, allows angular movements and other findings to be added. Charts may be compiled to denote primary and secondary dentition.

The extent of the history and examination varies between individuals, depending on their philosophy, their experience, expertise and specialty. A clinician rarely undertakes a complete history and examination of every system in a patient with clinical problems clearly confined to one particular area. A specialist who has seen a condition many times before can rapidly decide what is, and what is not, relevant.

The student will initially find it difficult to know what to leave out and will include a long list of irrelevant negatives on normal systems. This, however, is better than risking omission of relevant material. It is important that no clinician approaches a problem in a blinkered fashion, otherwise they will ask only leading questions and will miss other important abnormalities. The student should take the initial notes in rough and later streamline them for inclusion in a patient's record. Another problem is the use of abbreviations and shorthand. Each specialty produces its own language but the notes should always be meaningful to all health care workers who need to read them.

On completion of a history and examination, the clinician is in a position to assess the severity of the patient's problems and plan, with them, appropriate subsequent management. The time schedule will depend on the severity of the illness, and the patient's response to it and the advice given. The clinician will give particular emphasis to management of life threatening and treatable conditions.

Clinicians vary on how they record these recommendations in the clinical notes. A common practice after completion of the history and examination is to write a two or three sentence summary of the positive findings, followed by a provisional diagnosis, together with a list of proposed investigations and treatment. The disadvantages of this approach are that a diagnosis may not have been possible and there may be more than one problem deserving attention. An alternative 'problem orientated' approach lists the active and inactive problems encountered, and provides a management plan for each. Provided the positive plan is documented and initiated, either of these methods, or their modifications, is applicable.

Treatment regimes also need to be written out on drug and other therapeutic charts. Investigations must be checked and the results recorded. While the patient's condition is fluctuating a daily dated record of progress should be kept and any special events recorded in detail.

A note should be made of all procedures, including perioperative management; although it is common for there to be additional sheets for operative procedures and for the time spent in specialist units, such as intensive care. While in hospital, a progress note should be written at least weekly. A note should be made of the date and condition of a patient on discharge from hospital, including the medication prescribed and the proposed follow-up date. This information and a brief summary of the admission is taken by the patient, or posted directly, to the general practitioner to ensure continuity of care.

The condition on subsequent follow-up examination in hospital or at home should further be recorded. The extent to which the full history and examination are repeated depends on whether new problems arise or whether there is a long time interval between follow-up visits.

Neonatal Screening

Approximately 2% of newborn babies have life threatening congenital defects, some being incompatible with further existence. At birth the first priority is to ensure normal respiration and to institute immediate management of existing or suspected illness. The latter may be represented by abnormalities of colour (pallor, jaundice, cyanosis), posture (hyper/hypotonia), abnormal movement and an abnormal cry (altered pitch and volume). Urine and meconium are usually passed within 24 hours. The umbilical cord remnant separates about the seventh day. A routine examination is undertaken within 48 hours, to identify minor as well as obvious abnormalities. The following list considers the areas of examination and the abnormalities being sought:

Weight and length are related to dates: intrauterine malnutrition

Head circumference/fontanelles: micro/hydrocephalus

Facial features: Down's and other syndromes

Eyes: corneal and lens opacities, glaucoma

Mouth/jaw: cleft lip/palate, micro/macrognathia

Chest: congenital heart and lung disease

Abdomen: ventral and inguinal herniae, abdominal masses (renal, bladder)

Perineal: imperforate anus, genital abnormalities

Femoral pulses: coarctation of the aorta

Back: spina bifida, dermal sinus

Hips: congenital dislocation (of hip)

Limbs: abnormal length, abnormal number or conjoined digits, talipes, palmar creases of Down's syndrome

Altered reflexes: Moro, rooting, palmar grasp, stepping, placing, Babinski.

Milestones

Age in months	Posture and manipulation	Vision, hearing and speech	Behaviour
3	Raises head, holds head when held sitting	Watches moving object at 15cm, quietens to listen to sounds, coos	Smiles appropriately
6	pulls self to sit up, takes weight on legs when held, palmar grasp, puts objects into mouth	watches moving object at 2m, localises sound from each side at 45cm, double syllables	friendly to strangers
9	crawls, bounces when held standing, scissor grasp, transfers objects between hands	looks for objects, rapid localisation of sound at 90cm, tuneful babbling	apprehensive of strangers, chews solids
12	walks around furniture and when hands are held, pincer grasp	babbles incessantly, first words	understands simple commands cooperates with dressing
18	walks alone, builds three brick tower, scribbles	several words	demanding, drinks from cup with two hands
24	walks upstairs and runs, builds six brick tower	simple phrases	uses spoon, indicates toilet needs

Glossary

Abscess   A collection of pus circumscribed in a cavity produced by tissue disintegration and displacement.

Acanthocytosis   A condition of the blood in which there are intrinsically abnormal erythrocytes having an unusual distorted, crenated or thorny appearance when examined in wet preparations and films.

Accommodation   The mechanism by which the focus of the eye is shortened through contraction of the ciliary muscle, increasing the convexity of the lens.

Achalasia   1. Failure of relaxation in an opening of the body such as the oesophagus.   2. So-called cardiospasm.

Achondroplasia   A hereditary disease of the skeleton in which there is faulty endochondral ossification, resulting in dwarfism.

Acidosis   An increase in the $[H^+]$ in body fluids above the normal range. Usually defined as a decrease in pH of the blood below 7.36. It may be confined to a fluid compartment.

Acquired Immunodeficiency Disease (AIDS)   Viral infection producing a defect in cell-mediated immunity resulting (in the later stages of the disease) in opportunistic infections and uncommon malignancies.

Acromegaly   A chronic disease due to increased growth hormone. It is characterized by gradual enlargement of the hands and feet and of the bones of the head and chest.

Addison's Disease   A disease due to atrophy or tuberculosis of the adrenal cortex leading to deficiency or absence of cortisol.

Adenoid   1. Having resemblance or relating to a gland.   2. Resembling or relating to lymphoid tissue.

Agnosia   In this condition there is inability to recognize objects and lack of the perceptive faculty in general. Agnosia is found in relation with the senses: auditory agnosia, gustatory agnosia, olfactory agnosia, visual agnosia and tactile agnosia.

Agraphia   A special form of apraxia in which there is a loss, or complete absence, of the ability to express ideas in a written form.

Alexia   1. Lack of ability, because of a disease of the brain, to understand printed words, although they are visible.   2. Lack of ability, because of disease of the brain, to read aloud.

Allergy   An imprecisely used synonym for hypersensitivity, usually used of immediate hypersensitivity.

Amnesia   Loss of memory of varying degree attributable to organic or psychological causes.

Anaemia   A condition of the blood in which there are quantitative and qualitative changes in the red cells (erythrocytes) and haemoglobin in the circulating blood and bone marrow; there may also be a reduction in the total amount of blood (*oligohaemia*) temporarily, as in a severe acute haemorrhagic condition.

Anacrotic Pulse   Abnormality of the pulse wave which shows a small wave on the ascending limb.

Anaphylaxis   A condition of hypersensitivity to certain foreign proteins, resulting from the liberation of histamine.

Anarthria   The loss of the ability to articulate words.

Aneurysm   A localized dilatation of the walls of a blood vessel, usually an artery, due to weakening through infection, injury, degenerative conditions or congenital defects.

Angina   A tight precordial strangling or oppressive sensation, discomfort, or pain, caused by coronary artery disease.

Angioma   A benign tumour composed of blood or lymphatic vessels.

Angioplasty   Radiological dilatation of a diseased artery.

Anisocytosis   An abnormal condition in which the erythrocytes are not all of the same size.

Ankylosis   Complete immobility of a joint resulting from pathological changes in that joint or of the structures associated with it.

Aphasia   Inability to produce or to understand spoken or written speech, due to pathological interference with the speech centre or speech region of the brain.
   Global Aphasia A form of aphasia involving all the functions of speech.
   Jargon Aphasia A form of aphasia in which several words are expressed in a jumbled form as one word, with wrong placing of accent.
   Nominal Aphasia Inability to name people or objects.
   Receptive Aphasia Sensory aphasia. A type of aphasia which is the result of injury to the receptive mechanism; the meaning of words both written and spoken is not understood.

Apraxia   A disorder of voluntary movement characterized by the inability to perform, command or imitate a familiar action, the nature of which is understood, in the absence of severe inco-ordination or paralysis of the parts concerned.

Areflexia   A condition in the which the reflexes cannot be elicited, or are absent, generally as a result of breakdown in the reflex arc.

Arrhythmia   A disturbance of cardiac rate and rhythm.

Arteriography   The visualization of arteries by means of x-rays after injection of radio-opaque material.

Arteriosclerosis   See *Atheroma*.

Arteriovenous Malformation   Congenital abnormality of vascular development resulting in a focal or regional overgrowth.

Ascites   An abnormal accumulation of fluid in the peritoneal cavity.

Aspiration   The act of withdrawal by suction of fluid, gas or tissue from any part of the body.

Asthma   A syndrome characterized by paroxysmal attacks of dyspnoea of expiratory type.

Ataxia   Loss of control over the voluntary movements of everyday life, which depend upon the various groups of muscles involved in being completely balanced with each other.

Atheroma   The process affecting blood vessels involving the formation of sub-intimal plaques which start as lipid (cholesterol) deposits and which later become fibrotic or calcified. The surface may ulcerate and superimposed thrombosis occur. It is the commonest form of arterial disease.

Atheromatous   Affected with or pertaining to atheroma.

Athetosis   Slow, writhing involuntary movements mainly affecting the distal segments of the upper limbs. Most commonly occurring as a form of infantile cerebral palsy but also in hemiplegia from any cause. Bilateral athetosis is a juvenile form of dystonic movement disorder.

Athetoid   Affected with or resembling athetosis.

Atrial Septal Defect   A defect in the interatrial (interauricular) septum between the two atria of the heart. Consequently there is a left-to-right shunt which increases the amount of blood in the right side of the heart and in the pulmonary artery.

Atrophy   1. Wasting of a tissue or organ.   2. A condition of general malnutrition, from whatever cause, the signs of which are wasting or shrinking of the tissues of the whole body or of a part of it.

Auscultation   The art of listening to and interpreting the meaning of sounds produced within the body.

Autopsy   Post-mortem examination of a body, including its organs, in order to establish the cause of death; necropsy.

Babinski Response   Babinski reflex; the extensor plantar response which occurs in pyramidal-tract disease: on stroking the lateral aspect of the sole of the foot there is spontaneous dorsiflection of the great toe with 'fanning' of the other toes.

Bacteriology   The science that deals with bacteria.

Benign   1. Of a disease, mild or non-malignant; favouring recovery. 2. Of a neoplasm, unlikely to recur.

Biopsy   Examination, for purposes of diagnosis, tissues cut from the living body. These may be normal or diseased.

Bjerrum Screen   A black cloth screen, usually 2m square, with a central small white disc for fixation, placed 2m from the patient and well illuminated. Round white or coloured targets varying from 1 to 40mm are moved over this area and the central field of vision thus minutely investigated. It is a form of perimetry.

Blood Dyscrasia   A developmental disorder of the blood.

Borborygmus   The rumbling or gurgling sound made by movement of flatus in the intestines.

Bovine Cough   A prolonged and wheezing cough associated with paralysis of the recurrent laryngeal nerve.

Bradycardia   Slowing of the heart rate.

Bronchiectasis   Dilatation of a bronchus or bronchi, secondary to structural changes in the bronchial walls which are predominantly inflammatory in origin.

Bronchitis   An inflammation of the mucous membrane of the larger and medium-sized bronchi.

Bronchoscopy   The examination of the inside of a bronchial tube with a bronchoscope.

Brucellosis   Infection with a coccobacillus, usually acquired from the milk of farm animals.

Bruit A sound heard on auscultation, particularly an abnormal sound. It usually refers to sounds over a large artery, but may be used as a synonym for murmur, e.g. the systolic bruit of mitral disease.

Bryant's Triangle A triangle marked on the skin of a supine patient by dropping a vertical line from the anterior superior iliac spine to a horizontal directed cranially from the upper margin of the greater trochanter. It is used to detect a shortening of the femoral neck.

Bulbar Palsy Palsy due to degeneration of the nuclear cells of the lower cranial nerves; it is associated with progressive muscular atrophy.

Bursa A closed cavity in the connective tissue between two structures which move relative to one another, e.g. between a tendon and an adjacent bone.

Cachexia An extreme state of general ill-health with malnutrition, wasting, anaemia, and muscular weakness.

Calcaemia Pertaining to the amount of calcium in the blood: hyper- (excess) or hypo- (reduced).

Calculus A solid pathological concretion, usually of inorganic matter in a matrix of protein and pigment, formed in any part of the body, especially in reservoir organs and their passages.

Campbell de Morgan Spot A small red vascular haemangioma usually noted on the trunk, having no pathological significance.

Carcinoma A malignant epithelial tumour which tends to spread locally, and generally throughout the body, destroying normal tissues as it progresses and eventually proving fatal. It is most common after middle age.

Caries Tooth decay.

Cheyne-Stokes Breathing Cheyne-Stokes respiration; rhythmical waxing and waning of respiration, consisting of alternating periods of hyperpnoea (increased depth and rate of respiration), and apnoea (cessation of respiration). Respiration steadily increases in depth, then wanes, until finally it ceases entirely. After a few moments the cycle is repeated.

Chorea   Acute chorea; Sydenham's chorea. A disease chiefly affecting children and characterized by irregular involuntary movements of the limbs and face.

Choreiform   Describing the movements of chorea.

Cirrhotic Liver   A liver showing overgrowth of the supporting connecting tissue from whatever cause.

Cleft Lip   Hare-lip; A congenital malformation of the upper lip due to failure of fusion of the maxillary processes with the frontonasal process, frequently associated with cleft palate.

Clonus   A sign of increased reflex activity as in upper motor neuron lesions, characterized by repetitive muscular contraction induced by stretch.

Clubbing   A condition which affects the fingers and toes in many diseases of widely different aetiology. The ends of the fingers and toes show a characteristic deformity which is most easily detected in the fingers. The soft tissues are enlarged but the most outstanding feature of clubbing is seen in the nails, which are curved both laterally and longitudinally, presenting a bulbous, shiny appearance which varies from a slight departure from normal, as in the early stages of infective endocarditis, to the gross changes described as *drumstick* or *parrot's beak* in septic pulmonary disease or some congenital cardiac diseases. Clubbing of the fingers is most commonly found in 1) diseases of the lung such as bronchiectasis, cancer, septic diseases of the lung and the pneumoconioses; 2) infective endocarditis and some other cardiac conditions; 3) steatorrhoea, ulcerative colitis, subphrenic abscess and polycythaemia.

Coarctation of the Aorta   Narrowing of the lumen of the aorta, due to congenital maldevelopment.

Colic   A severe spasmodic griping pain which increases in intensity to a climax then remits for a short period and returns with equal intensity. Arises from powerful contractions of a muscular tube such as the intestine or ureter.

Colonoscopy   Examination of the colon by means of a colonoscope.

Coma The state of complete loss of consciousness from which the patient cannot be roused by an ordinary external stimulus; conjunctival and pupillary reflexes are absent and deep reflexes are usually abolished.

Consensual A term descriptive of reflex excitement of one part as the result of stimulation of another, usually the conjugate part, e.g the pupils of both eyes react alike although stimulation is applied to only one.

Consolidation The process of being converted into a firm mass, as occurs in the lung when the alveoli fill with exudate in cases of pneumonia.

Contracture 1. A prolonged reversible contraction of skeletal muscle which may affect only a part, and in which no wave-like action potentials occur. 2. Deformity due to shortening of muscle, usually the result of fibrosis.

Corneal Opacity An opaque or non-transparent area or spot within the cornea.

Craniotomy 1. An operation on the skull. 2. The cutting away of a part of the skull.

Crepitus 1. The sound of two rough substances being rubbed together. 2. A crepitant râle. 3. The sound produced when pressure is applied to tissues filled with gas or air, e.g. in subcutaneous emphysema.

Crohn's Disease An inflammatory lesion of the intestines of unknown cause.

Cushing's Disease An endocrine abnormality characterized by obesity of the trunk, purple striae on the abdomen and flanks, hypertension, polycythaemia, osteoporosis and glycosuria in either sex and by hypertrichosis, excessive bruising and amenorrhoea in women.

Cyanosis A blue appearance of the skin and mucous membranes, which may be general but is most prominent in the extremities, hands and feet, and in superficial highly vascular parts such as the lips, cheeks and ears. It is due to deficient oxygenation of the blood in the small blood vessels and capillaries, and depends upon the absolute amount of reduced haemoglobin present.

Cyst   A cavity lined by a well-defined epithelium, fibrous tissue, or degenerating, inflamed or neoplastic tissue.

CVP   Central Venous Pressure.

Demyelination   The removal or destruction of the myelin of nerve tissue.

Diabetes   1. Without qualification the word is usually taken to mean *diabetes mellitus*.   2. Any one of a group of diseases in which there is polyuria and/or an error of metabolism, especially of carbohydrate metabolism.

Diabetes Mellitus   A disease, of which there are several forms, characterized by a high-fasting blood sugar, an exaggerated rise in the blood sugar after the ingestion of glucose and a failure of the blood sugar to return in a normal time to normal values.

Diastole   The period of the cardiac cycle from the closure of the aortic and pulmonary valves to the beginning of the next ventricular contraction. The period when the heart fills with blood and dilates.

Dislocation   Displacement of one part upon another; usually confined to the abnormal displacement of one bone upon another at a joint.

Divarication   Separating or stretching.

Diverticulum   A pouch or cul-de-sac of a hollow organ.

Down's Syndrome   Mongolism; associated with an error in chromosomal separation during the formation of the germ cells.

Duodenal Ulcer   A peptic ulcer situated in the duodenum usually near the pylorus.

Dupuytren's Contracture   Palmar contraction; a thickening of the palmar fascia causing slow flexion deformity of the fingers and usually mainly affecting the ring and little fingers.

DVT   Deep Vein Thrombosis.

Dysarthria   Difficulty in articulating words caused by disease of the central nervous system.

Dysdiadochokinesis   The slow, clumsy and irregular performance of alternating movements of a limb that characterizes the presence of a lesion of the cerebellum.

Dyskinesia   1. Impairment of voluntary motion, causing movements that are incomplete or only partial.   2. Involuntary movement (incorrect usage).

Dysmenorrhoea   Pain occurring in the back and lower abdomen at or about the time of menses.

Dyspareunia   Difficulty or pain on intercourse.

Dysphagia   Difficulty in swallowing.

Dysphasia   Difficulty in speaking, with inability to co-ordinate words and arrange them in correct order.

Dyspnoea   The subjective feeling of discomfort or distress which occurs when the need for increased pulmonary ventilation has reached the point of obtruding unpleasantly into consciousness.
  Paroxysmal Dyspnoea Episodic dyspnoea occurring at rest and frequently during the night, secondary to left heart failure.

Dysuria   A condition in which the passing of urine is painful or difficult.

Ectopic   An organ or substance not in its proper position, or of a pregnancy, (ectopic gestation) occurring elsewhere than in the cavity of the uterus.

Eczema   A non-contagious inflammatory disease of the skin.

Effusion   1. Escape of fluid, e.g. blood, on account of rupture or of exudation through the walls of a vessel.   2. A fluid discharge, often into a cavity, e.g. a joint or a pleural cavity.

Ehlers-Danlos Syndrome   Congenital disease with increased elasticity of the skin and increased laxity of the joints, fragility of the skin, pseudotumours resembling haemangiomata and reduction of subcutaneous fat; occasionally subcutaneous nodules are present.

Electrocardiogram   ECG; a record of the electrical potentials generated by the activation process of the muscle of the heart.

Embolism   The sudden blocking of a blood vessel, usually an artery, by fragments of a blood clot, or by clumps of bacteria or other foreign bodies introduced into the circulation.

Emphysema   A condition in which the alveoli of the lungs are dilated.

Enophthalmos   Recession of the eyeball into the cavity of the orbit.

Epididymo-orchitis   A condition of inflammation involving both the epididymis and the testis.

Epilepsy   An affection of the nervous system characterized by recurrent paroxysmal symptoms, the epileptic fit, resulting from excessive or disordered discharge of cerebral neurons.

Epistaxis   Bleeding from the nose.

Erythema   Redness of the skin due to hyperaemia.

Erythema Ab Igne   Erythema in a reticular pattern due to exposure to heat. It is usually seen on the antero-lateral surface of the lower legs, from sitting in front of a fire, or on the abdomen where a hot water bottle has been applied for pain relief.

External Auditory Meatus   A sinuous channel connecting the auricle with the tympanum and closed at its inner end by the tympanic membrane, set in an oblique plane so that the anterior wall and floor are longer than the posterior wall and roof.

Exophthalmos   Prominence or protrusion of the eyeball.

Faeculent   Of a faecal nature.

Fallot's Tetralogy   Tetralogy indicates that a combination of four anomalies are found: 1. stenosis of the pulmonary artery; 2 a defect in the interventricular septum; 3. an aorta which, instead of arising solely from the left ventricle, 'overrides' the interventricular septum and thus receives blood from the right and left ventricle, i.e. there is a right-to-left shunt; 4. an enlarged right ventricle.

Fasciculation   1. The process of formation of fasciculi.   2. Arrangement in the form of clusters of bundles   3. Spontaneous contraction of bundles of muscle fibres visible through the skin.   4. Fibrillary twitching of voluntary muscles seen, for example, after the injection of a depolarizing myoneural blocking agent.

Fibrillation   1. The condition of being fibrillar or fibrillated. 2. Spontaneous contraction of individual muscle fibres; a sign of denervation.
   Auricular: spontaneous contraction of auricular muscle.

Fibroid   1. Resembling fibrous tissue or a fibrous structure.   2. A fibroma, myoma, fibromyoma, or leiomyofibroma especially of the uterus.

Fissure   A groove, cleft or furrow; a sulcus; a natural one due to infolding during development, e.g. between the cerebral convolutions, or a pathological one, e.g. the partial fracture of a bone.

Fit   A colloquial term applied to many forms of sudden disorder of function, especially of consciousness, e.g. fainting fit (syncope), apoplectic fit (stroke). Medically now almost always confined to the paroxysmal symptoms of various forms of epilepsy.

Flutter   A tremulousness.

Foerster's cutaneous numeral test   A clinical test of topognostic sensibility: the patient closes his eyes and a number is traced out with a blunt instrument upon his skin. Repeated failure to recognize numerals so traced indicates impairment of the finer elements of sensation (tactile discrimination and topognostic sensibility) in the skin area tested and usually means a lesion in the sensory cortex or in the posterior column of the spinal cord.

Fracture   1. To break a structure, especially a bone.   2. A break or interruption in the continuity of a bone.

Galactorrhoea   1. Spontaneous secretion and discharge of milk after the period of nursing is over.   2. An excessive flow of milk.

Gallstone   A concretion which may form in the gall bladder or bile duct. Its composition most commonly is of cholesterol.

Gangrene   Necrosis or putrefaction of tissue due to cutting off the blood supply; the term usually refers to skin necrosis, but it may also occur in the bowel.

Gastroduodenoscopy   Inspection of the stomach and duodenum by means of a fibreoptic endoscope, normally passed through the mouth.

Glands of Montgomery   Small prominences, sebaceous glands, in the areola of the breast which become more marked in pregnancy.

Glaucoma   A term signifying increased intra-ocular pressure and its consequences.

Goitre   An enlargement of the thyroid gland; it is usually taken to mean a visible enlargement.

Graphaesthesia   The ability to recognize letters or figures traced on the skin by blunt pressure, as in Foerster's cutaneous numeral test.

Haematuria   The presence of blood in the urine.

Haemoglobinopathy   A disease of the blood associated with the presence of an abnormal haemoglobin in the red blood cells.

Haemolysis   The release of haemoglobin from the red cells as a result either of osmotic effects or of the breaking-up or laking of the red blood cells.

Haemoptysis   The expectoration of bright red blood from the lungs or bronchi and trachea.

Haemorrhage   Bleeding; the escape of blood from any part of the vascular system.
  Splinter Haemorrhage: Linear haemorrhage under the nails, seen in malignant endocarditis.

Haemorrhoid   A swelling at the anal margin; a pile.

Halitosis   Fetid or offensive breath.

Hashimoto's Disease   Struma lymphomatosa, a chronic thyroiditis associated with auto-immune antibodies to thyroxin in the blood serum.

Heart Block   A condition in which the transmission of impulses from the sinu-atrial node through the atria, atrioventricular node and bundle of His to the ventricles is delayed or interrupted in some part of its course.

Hepatitis   Inflammation of the liver.

Hepatocellular Dysfunction   *Hepatocellular:* relating to or having an effect on liver cells.

Hepatoma   A combined adenomatous and carcinomatous neoplasm originating in the hepatic parenchyma.

Hepatosplenomegaly   A enlarged condition of the liver and the spleen.

Horner's Syndrome   Slight enophthalmos, meiosis, and slight ptosis, with narrowing of the palpebral fissure, with sometimes decrease of sweating, vasodilatation of the conjunctival, retinal and facial vessels, and rise in the skin temperature: due to damage of the cervical sympathetic chain.

Howell-Jolly Bodies   Spherical, eccentrically-placed granules or nuclear remnants about 1μm in diameter, occasionally seen in red blood corpuscles, usually very numerous in haemolytic or toxic anaemias and after splenectomy.

Hydrocele   A circumscribed collection of fluid, particularly a collection of fluid in the tunica vaginalis testis.

Hydrocephalus   An abnormal increase of cerebrospinal fluid within the skull.

Hyperaemia   An excess of blood in any part of the body.
   Reactive Hyperaemia: Increased blood flow after temporary ischaemia.

Hyperaesthesia   Excessive sensitiveness of the skin, due to local causes or to peripheral nerve damage.

Hyperdynamic   Abnormally great muscular or nervous activity; extreme functional energy.

Hyperkalaemia   An excess of potassium in the blood.

Hyperkeratinisation   The horny thickening of the epithelium, e.g. of palms and soles, which is characteristic of chronic arsenical poisoning or due to vitamin A deficiency.

Hyperkinesia   A condition in which there is abnormally great strength of movement, as in muscular spasm.

Hyperparathyroidism   Abnormally increased activity of the parathyroid glands due to a neoplasm or to hyperplasia.

Hypertension   High arterial blood pressure usually in the systemic arterial circulation. It may also be in the pulmonary arteries, secondary to lung disease, or in the portal venous system, due to liver disease.

Hypertonia   1. Excessive tension, as of arteries or muscles.   2. Excessive activity, as of muscles.   3. A state of increased intra-ocular tension.

Hypertrophic Obstructive Cardiomyopathy (HOCM)   Congenital overgrowth of cardiac muscle particularly affecting the left ventricle and interventricular septum.

Hypertrophic Pulmonary Osteoarthropathy   Proliferative periostitis at the distal end of long bones, particularly of the wrist and ankle, always associated with gross clubbing, and usually indicative of carcinoma of the bronchus.

Hypertrophy   An increase in the number or size of the cells of which a tissue is composed as a result of increase in function of that tissue.
   Ventricular Hypertrophy: Enlargement of the heart muscle of the ventricles as a result of valvular disease or hypertension.

Hypocalcaemia   A low calcium content of the blood.

Hypocarbia Low carbon dioxide on blood gas analysis.

Hypoglycaemia A low blood sugar concentration.

Hypokalaemia A low blood potassium.

Hyporeflexia A condition in which there is only weak reflex action.

Hypothyroidism A condition caused by under-activity of the thyroid gland; thyroid deficiency.

Hypotonia 1. Lessened tone or tension, generally, or applied to any body structure. 2. Arterial hypotension. 3. Deficient intra-ocular tension.

Hypoxaemia A condition in which the blood contains too little oxygen.

Hypoxia A supply of O_2 to the tissues which is inadequate to maintain normal tissue respiration.

Immunization The production of immunity by specific means: this may be the production of active immunity by the injection (or other modes of administration) of antigenic materials, or passive immunity by the injection of antibodies, in serum or serum fractions, developed in human or animal.

Impaction 1. One fragment of bone driven into another. 2. Faeces firmly lodged in the bowel. 3. Wedged close together, as with unerupted teeth.

Imperforate Anus An anus where there is no opening from the rectum to the exterior owing to failure of the cloacal membrane to break down.

Impotence Inability to perform the sexual act (in contradistinction to sterility: inability to reproduce), owing to failure of the reflex mechanism.

Infarct A wedge-shaped area of dead tissue, with or without haemorrhage, produced by an obstruction of an end artery.

Infection The invasion of the body by pathogenic or potentially pathogenic organisms, and their subsequent multiplication in the body.

Inflammation   The reactive state of hyperaemia and exudation from its blood vessels, with consequent redness, heat, swelling, and pain, which a tissue enters in response to physical or chemical injury or bacterial invasion.

Intermittent Claudication   A syndrome which is one of the earliest signs of partial impairment of the arterial flow. Severe pain in the legs, tension and weakness after the patient has been walking for a certain distance occur, and the symptoms increase as walking proceeds until further progress is impossible. After a short rest, during which the symptoms cease, walking becomes possible again.

Intracranial Pressure   The pressure in the subarachnoid space between the skull and the brain; if there is free circulation of the fluid and the patient is recumbent this is the same as the cerebrospinal pressure as measured by lumbar puncture.

Intubation   1. The therapeutic use of a tube.   2. The introduction of a tube into the larynx through the glottis in order to permit air to pass in and out, as in anaesthesia, diphtheria or in oedema of the glottis.   3. Catheterization.

Ipsilateral   Occurring or located on the same side; denoting symptoms of paralysis or other disorder which are present on the same side as the cerebral lesion which has caused them.

Ischaemia   Insufficient blood supply to a part of the body relative to the local needs, usually the result of disease of the blood vessels supplying the parts affected.

Ishihara Chart   Ishihara's Colour-Vision Test; the patient is shown a number of plates made up of coloured circular dots. In each plate a number is picked out in dots of one colour with a background of a confusion colour. The patient with normal colour vision reads the number correctly, while the colour-blind patient sees another number.

Jaundice   Icterus; a syndrome characterized by an excess of bile pigment in the blood (hyperbilirubinaemia) and consequent deposition of bile pigment in the skin, sclera, mucous membranes, and generally in the urine.

Keratosis A lesion of the skin or of a mucocutaneous junction caused by many different aetiological factors and essentially degenerative in type. The epidermis is usually atrophic and shows hyperkeratosis and parakeratosis. Vascular dilatation and degenerative changes are often to be seen in the corium and the condition must often be regarded as premalignant.

Ketosis The presence of excessive quantities of ketone bodies in the tissues.

Klinefelter's Syndrome Congenital defect characterized by testicular dysgenesis with aspermatogenesis associated with a high output of gonadotrophins and sometimes gynaecomastia.

Koilonychia A condition in which the sides of the nail are raised and there is a concavity in the centre of the nail; spoon nail.

Koplik Spots Bluish-white specks, usually surrounded by a red ring, seen on the mucous membrane of the mouth in measles.

Kussmaul Breathing Extreme hyperpnoea; seen in diabetic coma.

Kviem Test A test for sarcoidosis, by the intradermal injection of material from a gland of a person known to have Boeck's sarcoid.

Kyphosis Spinal curvature in which the concavity of the curve is in a forward direction, generally in the thoracic region.

Laparoscopy The act or process of examining the peritoneal cavity and its contents by means of a laparoscope.

Laparotomy An exploratory incision through the abdominal wall.

Leukaemia A disease of the leucocytopoietic tissues, first in the bone marrow and then affecting the blood and other organs.
Acute Lymphoblastic Leukaemia: An acute leukaemia with lymphoblasts or lymphocytes as the main cells concerned.
Myeloblastic Leukaemia: Chronic myelosis, a chronic form of leukaemia with mild to very great splenomegaly and hepatomegaly, and usually of relatively slow progress (3–16 years); it usually shows a very high myeloid leucocytosis in blood and bone marrow when first diagnosed.

Leukoplakia   A chronic inflammatory lesion resulting in the formation of smooth, dry, white, thickened patches in the mucous membrane, especially the mouth, where it may occur on the tongue, inside of the cheeks, or gums.

Lordosis   Spinal curvature in which the convexity of the curve is in a forward direction, generally in the lumbar region.

Lymphadenitis   Inflammation of the lymph nodes.

Lymphadenopathy   Any morbid condition of the lymph glands.

Lymphoma   A general term comprising tumours, and conditions allied to tumours, arising from some or all of the cells of lymphoid tissue.

Macrocytosis   Macrocythaemia; the presence of macrocytes in the blood.

Macrognathia   A condition in which the jaw is larger than normal.

Malabsorption   1. Defective absorption of fluids or of any other nutritive substances.   2. Defective anabolism.

Malgaigne's Bulge   Bulge along the line of the inguinal canal due to muscle laxity, independent of the presence of an inguinal hernia.

Malignant   1.Threatening life or tending to cause death; the opposite of benign.   2. Virulent.   3. Recurrent, even after careful extirpation; this is in special reference to neoplasms.

Mammography   The study of the mammary gland by a specialized soft-tissue radiographic technique without injection of a radio-opaque contrast medium.

Mantoux/Heaf Test   An intracutaneous injection of tuberculin to assess immunity to tuberculosis.

Marfan's Syndrome   A congenital mesodermal disturbance of hereditary nature, with variable clinical presentation. Common features are tall stature, increased span, long thin digits (arachnodactyly), subluxation of the lens of the eyes, weakness of the arterial walls leading to dissecting aneurysms or rupture of the aorta, or globular dilatation of the aortic root with aortic regurgitation.

McMurray Test   Test to demonstrate damaged knee cartilages.

Meconium   The first matter, dark green in colour and consisting of bile, mucoid debris, and epithelial elements, discharged from the bowels of a newborn infant.

Mediastinoscopy   Examination of the mediastinum through a small supersternal incision by means of an endoscope.

Meiosis   The process of cell division which results in the production of haploid cells from diploid parents; reduction division. In almost all animals meiosis takes place during gametogenesis.

Menarche   The establishment of the menses.

Menopause   Literally, the cessation of spontaneous menstrual periods. The period at which normal menstrual life ceases; the climacteria or change of life.

Mesothelioma   A malignant tumour of the mesothelium of the pleura, pericardium or peritoneum, diagnostic of exposure to asbestos.

Metastasis   The transfer of disease from its primary site to distant parts of the body by way of natural passages, blood vessels, lymphatics, or direct continuity.

MI   Myocardial infarction.

Microcephalus   A person with an unusually small size of head; generally a microcephalic idiot.

Microcytosis   Microcythaemia. The presence of an excess of microcytes in the blood.

Micrognathia   Undersize of the jaw; particularly applied to the mandible.

Mikulicz's Syndrome   Bilateral symmetrical enlargement of the lacrimal and salivary glands. Now regarded to be of the same nature as Sjörgen's disease.

Moro Reflex   Startle reflex.

Mucocele   1. A mucous (gelatinous) polypus.   2. A dilated cavity containing an accumulation of mucoid substance.

Mucoid   Of the nature of mucus.

Mucopurulent   Composed of or containing mucus and pus.

Mucus   The viscous secretion of mucous membrane upon which it has a protective action. Its chief constituent is mucin.

Multiple Myeloma   Myelomatosis, a tumour arising from the bone marrow and most often affecting the flat bones.

Multiple Sclerosis   Disseminated, focal or insular sclerosis; the occurrence of patches of demyelination in the brain and spinal cord.

Murmur   A continuous sound; a bruit.
   Diastolic Murmur: A murmur occurring during the phase of ventricular diastole. When arising from the aortic or pulmonary valves it indicates valve incompetence, but if from the mitral or tricuspid valves, stenosis.
   Ejection Murmur: A murmur produced by the ejection of blood from either ventricle. It is usually harsh, best heard over the base of the heart and crescendo-decrescendo in form, starting very shortly after the first heart sound (immediately after an ejection sound if one is present).
   Mid-Systolic Murmur: A murmur occurring in the middle phase of cardiac systole.
   Pansystolic Murmur: A systolic murmur which occurs throughout the whole of systole; it usually also varies little in intensity or quality throughout its duration.
   Systolic Murmur: A murmur occurring during cardiac systole.

Myasthenia Gravis   Abnormal fatigability of the muscles due to impairment of conduction at the motor end-plate.

Myelodysplasia   Imperfect development of any portion of the spinal cord, in particular of the lower segments.

Myocardial Infarct   An infarct of the heart muscle due to inadequacy of blood supply which mostly commonly results from atheromatous disease of the coronary arteries, often with superimposed thrombotic occlusion of a vessel.

Myotonia   A difficulty or slowness in relaxing muscles after effort.

Myxoedema   A condition due to hypothyroidism, and characterized by mucoid infiltration of the skin and subcutaneous tissue, dryness of the skin, loss of hair, sensitivity to cold, mental dullness and a low basal metabolic rate.

Nausea   A feeling of sickness with the desire to vomit.

Nelaton's Line   A line joining the anterior superior iliac spine and the ischial tuberosity.

Neuritis   Inflammation of a nerve.

Neurosis   An illness of the personality, manifested as a functional derangement of the mind or body and differentiated in typical instances from psychosis by the retention of insight and by its less serious and less fundamental nature.

Nocturia   Getting up at night to pass urine.

Nodular   1. Resembling a node or nodule.   2. Studded with nodules.

Nodule   A small node, or aggregation of cells.

Oedema   The presence of excessive fluid in the intercellular tissue spaces of the body, due to increased transudation of fluid from the capillaries.
   Pulmonary Oedema: Oedema of the lungs, as in left-sided heart failure.

Oesophagoscopy   Visualising the interior of the oesophagus through an oesophagoscope.

Orthopnoea   A condition in which the patient can breathe comfortably only when sitting or standing erect.

Osler's Node   A small, raised, red, tender patch found on the pads of the fingers, and occasionally toes, in bacterial endocarditis. It is transient, and due to an infected cutaneous embolus.

Osteomalacia   Decalcification of the bones.

Osteitis Fibrosa   Parathyroid osteitis, a generalized rarefaction of bone, associated with cyst formation and replacement of bone by fibrous tissue, due to excessive parathyroid secretion.

Osteoarthritis   Chronic arthritis of a degenerative type, usually but not invariably associated with increasing age.

Osteoporosis   Rarefaction of bone.

Otitis Media   Inflammation of the middle ear.

Paget's Disease   1. Osteitis deformans.   2. A pseudo-eczematous condition of the nipple and areola, sometimes spreading to the surrounding skin, due to intra-epithelial spread of carcinoma cells from underlying breast ducts.

Pallor   Paleness.

Palpation   The method of physical examination in which the hands are applied to the surface of the body, so that by the sense of touch information is obtained about the condition of the skin, the underlying tissues, and organs.

Paracentesis   Surgical puncture, tapping, or needling of a cavity for evacuation of harmful content, or for removal of fluid material for diagnosis.

Paraesthesia   Numbness or tingling.

Paralysis   Loss of motor power due to a functional or organic disorder of neural or neuromuscular mechanisms; also called *palsy*.

Paraphimosis   A condition in which a phimosed prepuce is forcibly retracted behind the glans penis with the result that the tissues distal to the phimotic constriction becomes grossly oedematous owing to obstruction of their venous and lymphatic drainage.

Parkinsonism   Mask-like face, excessive salivation, loss of emotional and associated movements, static tremor inhibited by movement, and a festinant gait, due to a lesion of the globus pallidus and often the substantia nigra (the palaeostriatum).

Patent Ductus Arteriosis   Persistence of the normal fetal patency of the ductus arteriosus

Pathological   1. Relating to pathology.   2. Caused by or causing disease.   3. Indicating a disease state or condition.

Peau D'Orange   A condition caused by lymphatic oedema and characterized by the existence of dimples on the skin; typical of infiltrating carcinoma of the breast.

Pectus Carinatum   Pigeon chest.

Pectus Excavatum   Depressed anterior chest wall.

Percussion   The art of striking the thoracic or abdominal wall in order to produce sound vibrations from which the nature of the underlying structures can be deduced; it is based on the fact that when an elastic body capable of vibrating is struck, a sound will be produced.

Perforation   A hole made through the full thickness of a membrane or similar tissue, or through any substance.

Pericardial Rub   The rub which may occur with pericarditis.

Pericardial Tamponade   The compressive effect upon the heart of blood or fluid that has accumulated within the pericardial cavity.

Pericarditis   Inflammation of the pericardium, visceral, parietal, or both.

Peritoneal Rub   The rub which may occur with peritonitis.

Peritonism   The physical signs of abdominal tenderness, percussion rebound and guarding, characteristic of peritonitis.

Peritonitis   Inflammation of the peritoneum usually caused by bacterial infection.

Perseveration   The continuation or recurrence of an experience or activity, without the appropriate exciting stimulus.

Phaeochromocytoma   Tumour of the adrenal medulla giving rise to hypertension, hypermetabolism and hyperglycaemia with excessive production of catecholamines.

Philadelphia Chromosome   Ph Chromosome usually found in the bone marrow cells of patients with chronic myeloid leukaemia.

Phimosis   Narrowing of the preputial orifice so that the foreskin cannot be readily retracted. Usually congenital but may be acquired as a result of inflammatory fibrosis.

Pile   A haemorrhoid; a dilatation of a branch or branches of the haemorrhoidal veins. The term is also loosely applied to other anal swellings.

Pleurisy   Inflammation of the pleura.

Pleuroscopy   Examination of the cavity of the pleura through an incision in the wall of the thorax.

Pneumoperitoneum   Air or gas within the peritoneal cavity.

Pneumothorax   The presence of air or gas within the thorax, resulting in partial or complete collapse of the lung.

Poikilocytosis   A condition of the blood in which there are a large number of poikilocytes (an *erythrocyte*, usually bigger than normal and irregularly shaped), as in pernicious and certain other anaemias.

Polychromasia   Polychromatophilia. Variation in the haemoglobin content of the erythrocytes or the haemoglobinated normoblasts.

Polycythaemia   A condition in which there is an abnormal increase in the number of red cells in the circulating blood; there is usually an associated increase in the amount of cellular haemoglobin, in the volume of packed red cells and in blood viscosity.

Polyp   Polypus; a tumour with a stalk, arising from mucous membranes or the body surface.

Polypectomy The operation of removal of a polyp.

Polyuria Increase in the amount of urine excreted.

Priapism Persistent erection of the penis, as a rule not due to sexual desire but caused by penile injuries, stone in the urinary bladder, or lesions of the spinal cord. It also occurs in leukaemia.

Primary Biliary Cirrhosis Inflammation causing fibrosis with destruction of the bile ducts associated with deep jaundice, itching and high blood cholesterol level.

Proctoscopy Examination of the rectum by means of a proctoscope.

Pruritus Itching; a cutaneous subjective symptom producing a desire to scratch.

Pseudobulbar Palsy Bulbar symptoms due to supranuclear lesions.

Pseudocyst False cyst; a cyst-like space which develops in a tissue as the result of softening or necrosis of the tissue.

Psychosomatic Pertaining to the body-mind relationship.

Ptosis The prolapse or dropping of an organ; drooping of the upper eyelid, e.g. from paralysis of the third cranial nerve.

Pulsus Paradoxus Paradoxical pulse; a pulse which becomes smaller during inspiration.

Purulent 1. Characterized by the presence of pus. 2. Producing or containing pus; suppurative.

Pyrexia A fever; a condition characterized by fever.

Rash A cutaneous eruption.

Regurgitation 1. The return of swallowed food into the mouth. 2. The passive flow of liquid from the stomach or oesophagus into the pharynx in the absence of vomiting. 3. The return of blood through a heart valve.

Aortic Regurgitation: Aortic incompetence; failure of the aortic valves to close completely during ventricular diastole, with the result that the blood leaks back into the left ventricle.
Mitral Regurgitation: Mitral incompetence.

Resuscitation   1. The act or process of restoring to life or consciousness to anyone who is gravely collapsed or apparently dead.   2. The state of being resuscitated.   3. Revival.

Retention   The holding back in the body of substances which are normally excreted.

Rheumatic Fever   Acute rheumatism.

Rheumatism   A non-specific term for any painful condition arising in musculoskeletal tissues.

Rheumatoid Nodule   Rheumatic nodules. Aggregations of tissue cells of sufficient size to be detectable by the examining finger, situated in various soft tissues of the body, often over bony prominences.

Riedel's Lobe   A tongue-like downward projection of liver substance from the right lobe of the liver; a relatively common congenital abnormality.

Right Bundle Branch Block   Right Bundle Branch Heart Block. Failure of conduction of the excitatory impulse in the branch of the His bundle distributed within the right ventricle.

Rigidity   The state of stiffness and inflexibility.

Rinne's Test   In the diagnosis of deafness: a vibrating tuning fork is placed over the mastoid process; when it ceases to be heard, the prongs are held close to the external auditory meatus. A normal person should hear it for as long again. This is termed a *positive Rinne* response. If the sound is not heard when transferred to the meatus, the test is repeated, with the fork held first at the meatus and then over the mastoid process. If now the vibrations are heard by bone conduction, after hearing by aerial conduction has ceased, the result is know as a *negative Rinne* response.

Romberg's Sign   With the feet together the patient closes his eyes: swaying or falling is indicative of sensory ataxia due to loss of appreciation of position sense in the lower limbs.

Rombergism   The state of exhibiting a positive Romberg's sign.

Sarcoid   A systematic inflammatory disease of unknown aetiology, characterized by noncaseating granulomata.

Scar   Cicatrix; connective-tissue replacement of mesodermal or ectodermal tissue which has been destroyed by injury or disease.

Schistocytosis   A condition marked by the presence of numbers of schistocytes (fragmented or segmented red blood cells) in the blood.

Scoliosis   Lateral curvature of the spine.

Septicaemia   The severe type of infection in which the blood stream is invaded by large numbers of the causal bacteria which multiply in it and spread. It should be distinguished from bacteraemia in which organisms appear in the blood without the severe rapid generalization of infection characteristic of septicaemia.

Sigmoidoscopy   Inspection of the rectum and pelvic colon with a sigmoidoscope.

Sinus   An infected tract communicating with the skin or the lumen of a hollow viscus.

Sinus Arrhythmia   An irregularity of heart rhythm caused by changes in the vagus control of the sinu-atrial node during respiration.

Sinus Rhythm   The normal heart rhythm due to conduction of impulses from the sinu-atrial node to the atrioventricular node; the ventricles contract after each beat of the atria.

Sjögren's Syndrome   A syndrome characterized by deficient secretion of the lacrimal, salivary or other glands, giving rise to keratoconjunctivitis sicca, dry tongue and hoarse voice.

Snellen Chart   The test for distant visual acuity, consisting of black capital letters on a white board, properly illuminated.

Spasm   A sudden, powerful, involuntary contraction of muscle.

Spastic Hemiplegia   Hemiplegia with increased muscle tone.

Speculum   Any instrument used in the inspection of a tube or passage.

Spherocytosis   condition in which there are abnormally thick, almost spherical, red blood cells or spherocytes in the blood.

Sphincterotomy   Incision of a sphincter.

Spider Naevus   A small red, vascular dilatation from which capillaries radiate, and resemble a spider.

Spina Bifida   A defect in the development of the vertebral column in which there is a central deficiency of the vertebral lamina; the condition often affects several vertebrae, and is most common in the lumbar region. Variable protrusion of the meninges and of other contents of the spinal canal occurs through the gap, giving rise to a meningocele or a meningomyelocele.

Splitting   *Splitting of the heart sound:* a duplication of the first or second heart sounds. Splitting of the first heart sound may result from unequal closure of the mitral and tricuspid valves, as in bundle-branch block; splitting of the second is due to asynchronous closure of the pulmonary and aortic valves.

Sputum   The material expelled from the respiratory passages by coughing or clearing the throat.

Squint   A condition in which one eye deviates from the point of fixation.

Status Epilepticus   Repeated and prolonged epileptic seizures without recovery of consciousness between attacks.

Steatorrhoea   A condition in which an excess of split fat appears in the stools, as in coeliac disease.

Stenosis   The constriction or narrowing of an orifice or the lumen of a hollow or tubular organ.

Aortic Stenosis: Any form of narrowing of the left ventricular outflow.

Mitral Stenosis: Narrowing of the orifice of the mitral valve.

Pulmonary Stenosis: Any form of narrowing of the right ventricular outflow.

Pyloric Stenosis: Narrowing of the pyloric opening; it may be *congenital* (hypertrophic) due to thickened muscle in infants under six weeks old or *cicatricial,* usually due to ulcer or cancer.

Subvalvular Aortic Stenosis: Narrowing of the left ventricular outflow below the aortic valve.

Stereognosis   Ability to recognize the shape and character of an object by means of touch.

Stoma   1. A mouth-like opening, or pore, or communication between cavities.   2. An opening which leads into the gastro-intestinal tract from the outside or from one part of the intestine into another, e.g. gastrojejunal stoma, abdominal or perineal stoma.

Strangulated Hernia   Hernia, the contents of which have their vessels of supply constricted by the neck of the hernial sac or by the edges of the defect in the abdominal wall.

Subungual   Beneath a nail.

Suppuration   The production or exudation of pus.

Syncope   Transient loss of consciousness due to inadequate cerebral blood flow.

Synovitis   Inflammation of the synovial membrane of a joint. The condition is usually associated with an effusion of fluid within the synovial cavity.

Systolic   Relating to or resulting from a systole.

Tachycardia   Rapid action of the heart; there are wide limits of normality for adults, from 40 to 100 beats per minute.

Tachypnoea   Unduly rapid breathing.

Talipes   Club-foot; a deformity of the foot: the foot is of abnormal shape and is habitually held in an abnormal position.

Target Cell   An abnormal red cell which, when stained, appears to have the haemoglobin arranged as a circular central disc and an external concentric ring, thus giving the appearance of a target.

Telangiectasia   A condition of dilated capillary blood vessels, often multiple in character and forming angiomata.
  Hereditary Telangiectasia: Rendu-Osler-Weber disease, a hereditary disease characterized by recurrent bleeding from multiple telangiectases (dilated capillaries), usually in mucous membranes or skin, with normal platelet count, coagulation and bleeding times and clot retraction, but there is often a secondary anaemia.

Tenesmus   Straining; a painful endeavour to defaecate or urinate, or pain associated with defaecation or urination.

Tenosynovitis   Inflammation of a tendon sheath.

Thalassaemia   Cooley's anaemia, erythroblastic anaemia, Mediterranean disease, familial microcytic anaemia, target-cell anaemia: a chronic, progressive anaemia of congenital, familial, and racial incidence, showing splenomegaly, tone changes, mongoloid facies and typical target cells or thin, poorly staining red cells (leptocytes) in the circulating blood. The condition appears commonly in peoples from countries in a broad tropical belt extending from the Mediterranean basin through the Middle and Far East.

Thoracotomy   The operation of incising the wall of the thorax.

Thrill   1. A series of fine vibrations perceptible to the touch. They may also cause audible sound waves.   2. A palpable murmur; if sufficiently loud it will produce vibrations which can be felt through the skin.

Thromboembolic Disease   Thrombosis-producing embolism in the blood vessel.

Thrombosis   Intravascular coagulation during life, producing a thrombus.

Thyrotoxicosis   Graves' disease. Any toxic condition attributable to hyperactivity of the thyroid gland.

Tics   A coordinated repetitive movement, usually involving a number of muscles which follow their normal roles of prime mover, antagonist, and synergist. Tics commonly involve the face and shoulders, occur in people of neurotic disposition, and usually develop early in life.

Tinnel's Sign   Tingling sensation on percussion over a regenerating nerve ending.

Tinnitus   Subjective noise in the ear.

Tophi   A localized deposit of sodium biurate usually found in the region of joints in gouty patients. It generally occurs in cartilage or bone.

Traction   The act of pulling.

Tremor   A rhythmic, involuntary, purposeless, oscillating movement resulting from the alternate contraction and relaxation of opposing groups of muscles.

Trendelenburg Test   A tourniquet test to determine the integrity of the saphenous and deep veins of the lower limb.

Tricuspid Incompetence   Tricuspid insufficiency, tricuspid regurgitation; incompetence of the tricuspid valve.

Tuberculosis   The disease caused by infection with the *Mycobacterium tuberculosis.*

Tumour   A swelling.

Turner's Syndrome   A congenital abnormality, characterized by gonadal dysgenesis associated with webbing of the neck, short stature, and sometimes with coarctation of the aorta, cubitus valgus, scoliosis, and absence of upper lateral incisors.

Ulceration   The process of formation of an ulcer; a discontinuity of an epithelial covering.

Ulcerative Colitis   An ulcerative inflammation of the colon characterized by fever, anaemia and the passage of blood, mucus and pus from the bowels.

Uraemia   The condition which results from severe renal failure, and is associated with the retention of normal and abnormal metabolic products in the blood and disturbance of the acid-base ratio of the latter.

Urinalysis   The analysis of urine, chemically or bacteriologically.

Valgus   1. Displaced outwards from the central line of the body. 2. Talipes valgus   3. Genu valgus; knock-knees.

Valvotomy   Valvulotomy; the operation of splitting, with the finger or cutting with instruments, a stenotic valve, especially the mitral valve of the heart in mitral stenosis.

Varicocele   A swelling produced by varicosity of the veins of the *pampiniiform plexus,* i.e. a plexus of veins which lie in the spermatic cord anterior to the vas deferens.

Varicose Veins   Dilated, thin, tortuous superficial veins; usually of the lower limbs.

Varicosity   1. A morbid state marked by varices.   2. A varix or varicose vein.

Varus   1. Displaced inwards, towards the central line of the body. 2. Genu varus, or bow legs.   3. Inversion of the foot so that the weight is brought on to the outer part of the sole; talipes varus.

Ventricular Septal Defect   Two types exist: 1 A small defect, which may cause an abnormal cardiac murmur but which generally gives rise to no disability. This type is known as *maladie de Roger;* 2 A large defect in the interventricular septum, with a large left-to-right shunt. Like an interatrial septal defect, this leads to excess blood entering the right side of the heart and pulmonary circulation.

Vertigo   Giddiness, swimming in the head, a sense of instability, often with a sensation of rotation.

Viscus   A term applied to the internal organs of the body which are closely related to, or contained within the pleural, pericardial, or peritoneal cavities.

Vocal Resonance The sounds heard over the chest while a patient is speaking. A marked increase in the sound is called *bronchophony*.

Weber's Test In unilateral deafness: a vibrating tuning-fork placed on the vertex of the skull is normally heard in the midline. In unilateral conductive types of deafness, the vibrations are heard more intensely on the diseased side; in perceptive deafness, in the sound ear.

Whispering Pectoriloquy In which the whispered voice is conducted directly to the ear through the stethoscope in an area of the chest where it should not normally be heard. A more delicate sign than bronchophony but heard under the same physical conditions.

Xanthoma A fatty fibrous change in the skin associated with the formation of yellow or yellowish-brown plaques, nodules or tumours.

Zollinger-Ellison Syndrome A non-insulin-secreting adenoma of the islets of Langerhans associated with peptic ulceration.

Index

Hypertrophic obstructive cardiomy
  opathy (HOCM), 73, 78, 275
Hypertrophic pulmonary
  osteoarthropathy, 95, 275
Hypertrophy, 275
Hypocalcaemia, 275
Hypocarbia, 275
Hypochromia, 247
Hypoglycaemia, 240, 276
Hypokalaemia, 276
Hyporeflexia, 174, 276
Hypothalamo-pituitary/gonadal axis
  tests, 242
Hypothyroidism, 276
Hypotonia, 161, 276
Hypoxaemia, 276
Hypoxia, 276

Immunization, 276
Impaction, 276
Imperforate anus, 276
Impotence, 276
Infarct, 276
Infection, 276
Infective endocarditis, 69
Inflammation, 277
Inguinal hernia, 130–2, 133
Inguinal ligament, 130
Inguinal region, 130–1
Insulin test, 240
Intermittent claudication, 277
Interphalangeal joints, 206
Intestinal obstruction, 113, 115
Intracranial pressure, 277
Intradermal allergen test, 232
Intubation, 277
Ipsilateral, 277
Ischaemia, 277
Ischaemic limb, 89
Ishihara chart, 143, 277

Jaundice, 38, 277
Jaw protrusion, 150

Jejunal biopsy, 235
Joints, 183
  dislocation, 183
  position sense, 159
  subluxation, 183

Karyography (chromosome analysis),
  248–9
Keratosis, 278
Ketosis, 278
Kidney, 127
  mass, 127
  tenderness, 127
Klinefelter's syndrome, 248, 278
Knee joint, 214–8
  cruciate ligament function, 217
  effusion tests, 215–6
  loose bodies, 218
  meniscus, 218
Koilonychia, 278
Koplik spots, 278
Kussmaul breathing (air hunger), 95,
  278
Kveim test, 232, 278
Kyphosis, 94, 278

Lactose tolerance test, 236
Laparoscopy, 278
Laparotomy, 278
Larynx, 40
Left bundle branch block, 75
Left ventricular aneurysm, 73
Left ventricular hypertrophy, 73
Legal implications, 12–13
Leprosy, 155
Liver, 123
  cirrhotic, 267
  percussion, 117
  pressure over, 72
  pulsatility, 79
  Riedel's lobe, 123, 287
Liver function tests, 237–8
  alpha fetoprotein, 237

anti-nuclear factor, 237
biopsy, 238
serological markers, 237
synthetic, 237
ultrasonic scan, 237–8
Lordosis, 279
Lower motor neurone lesion, 179
Lumbar puncture, 244
Lumbar region, 126–7
Lundh test meal, 238
Lung:
  computerized axial tomography, 231
  crepitations, 79
  diffusion capacity, 230
  open biopsy, 230
  transbronchial biopsy, 230
  transthoracic biopsy, 230
  volume estimation, 229
Lung function tests, 229
Lymphadenitis, 279
Lymphadenopathy, 279
Lymph nodes:
  axillary, 51–3
  cervical, 48–50
  epitrochlear, 53
  inguinal, 53, 132
  para-aortic, 125
  popliteal, 53
  scalene, 97
  supraclavicular, 97
Lymphoma, 279

McMurray's test, 280
Macrocytosis, 279
Macrognathia, 279
Malabsorption, 279
Maladie de Roger, 293
Malgaigne's bulge, 131, 279
Mammography, 56, 279
Mantoux test, 232, 279
Marfan's syndrome, 31, 205, 279–80
Meconium, 280
Mediastinoscopy, 231, 280

Meiosis, 280
Memory disturbance, 141
Menarche, 280
Menopause, 280
Mental status, 25–7, 31, 142
Mesothelium, 280
Metacarpophalangeal joints, 205
  ulnar deviation, 183
Metastasis, 280
MI, 280
Microcephalus, 280
Microcytosis, 247, 280
Micrognathia, 280
Middle ear disease, 41
Midstream urine examination, 239
Mikulicz's syndrome, 42, 280
Milestones, 260
Mitral regurgitation, 73, 287
  murmur, 81
Mitral stenosis, 78, 290
  murmur, 81
Mitral valve prolapse, 78
  murmur, 81
Moles, 34
Moro reflex, 280
Motor function, 161–70
MRI angiography, 246
Mucocele, 281
Mucoid, 281
Mucopurulent, 281
Mucus, 281
Multiple myeloma, 184, 281
Multiple sclerosis, 244, 281
Mumps, 42
Murmurs, 281
Muscle, 161–70
  abnormal movements, 179
  atrophy, 184
  biopsy, 246
  bulk, 161, 162
  coordination, 171–3
  fascicular movements (flickering), 179
  observation, 161
  palpation, 161

Salivary glands, 42–3
Saphenous varix, 132
Sarcoid, 42, 232, 288
Scar, 288
Schistocytosis, 247, 288
Scoliosis, 94, 188, 288
Scrotum, 132–4
    invagination, 131
Sensation, somatic, 155–60
    inattention, 159
    light pressure, 155–6
    pain, 156
    steriognosis, 158
    temperature, 156–7
    touch, 155–6
    vibration, 157–8
Sensory evoked potentials, 244
Septicaemia, 288
Sigmoidoscopy, 235, 288
Sinus, 288
Sinus arrhythmia, 69–70, 288
Sinus rhythm, 70, 288–9
Shoulder girdle, 195–9
Sister Joseph's nodule, 114
Sjörgen's syndrome, 42, 289
Skills, 11–12
    clerical, 12
    communication, 11–12
    organisational, 12
    practical procedures, 13
Small bowel:
    biopsy, 235
    enema, 234
    function tests, 236
    pain, 111–2
Snellen chart, 143, 289
Spasm, 289
Spastic hemiplegia, 214, 289
Spasticity, 141–2
Speculum, 289
Spermatic cord, 133
Spherocytosis, 247, 289
Sphincterotomy, 289
Spider naevus, 289
Spina bifida, 289

Spine, 187–94
    curvatures, 187
    inspection, 187–8
    palpation, 188–94
Spirometry, 229
Spleen, 117, 124–5
Splenomegaly, 50
Splinter haemorrhages, 35, 69, 273
Splitting of heart sound, 289
Sputum, 33, 92, 95, 289
Squint, 290
Status epilepticus, 290
Steatorrhoea, 290
Stenosis, 290
Stereognosis, 158, 290
Sternoclavicular joint, 196
Stoma, 290
Strangulated hernia, 290
Stridor, 95
Stroke, 66
Subacromial bursa, 196
Sublingual glands, 42–3
Submandibular glands, 42–3
Subphrenic abscess, 111
Subungual, 290
Succussion splash, 128
Superior sulcus tumour, 95
Superior vena caval obstruction, 72
Suppuration, 290
Suprasternal notch, arterial impulse in,
    74
Surface membrane immunoglobulin
    (SmIG), 248
Syncope, 290
Synovial thickening, 184
Synovitis, 184, 290
Systolic, 291

Tachycardia, 291
Tachypnoea, 94, 291
Talipes, 291
Target cells, 247, 291
Taste testing, 149
Teeth, 108–9